KU-077-281

Epigraph

On this chill uncertain spring day, toward twilight, I have heard the first frog quaver from the marsh. That is a sound that Pharaoh listened to as it rose from the Nile, and it blended, I suppose, with his discontents and longings, as it does with ours. There is something lonely in that first shaken and uplifted trilling croak. And more than lonely, for I hear a warning in it, as Pharaoh heard the sound of plague. It speaks of the return of life, animal life, to the earth. It tells of all that is most unutterable in evolution – the terrible continuity and fluidity of protoplasm, the irrepressible forces of reproduction – not mystical human love, but the cold batrachian jelly by which we vertebrates are linked to the things that creep and writhe and are blind yet breed and have being. More than half it seems to threaten that when mankind has quite thoroughly shattered and eaten and debauched himself with his own follies, that voice may still be ringing out in the marshes of the Nile and the Thames and the Potomac, unconscious that Pharaoh wept for his son.

Donald Culross Peattie, *An Almanac for Moderns*
(Washington: The Limited Editions Club, 1938) p. 9.

v

The Politics of Emerging and Resurgent Infectious Diseases

Edited by

Jim Whitman
Lecturer, Department of Peace Studies
Bradford University

First published in Great Britain 2000 by
MACMILLAN PRESS LTD
Houndmills, Basingstoke, Hampshire RG21 6XS and London
Companies and representatives throughout the world

A catalogue record for this book is available from the British Library.

ISBN 0–333–69127–X

First published in the United States of America 2000 by
ST. MARTIN'S PRESS, LLC,
Scholarly and Reference Division,
175 Fifth Avenue, New York, N.Y. 10010

ISBN 0–312–22854–6

Library of Congress Cataloging-in-Publication Data
The politics of emerging and resurgent infectious diseases / edited by Jim
Whitman.
    p.   cm.
Includes bibliographical references and index.
ISBN 0–312–22854–6 (cloth)
1. Epidemiology. 2. Epidemics—Political aspects. I. Whitman, Jim.
RA651 .P66   2000
614.4'2—dc21

99–058996

Selection, editorial matter and Chapter 1 © Jim Whitman 2000
Chapter 2 © Manuel Carballo 2000
Chapter 3 © Debarati Guha-Sapir 2000
Chapter 4 © Publications Scientifiques, Institut Pasteur 2000
Chapter 5 © Kraig Klaudt 2000
Chapter 6 © Michael J. Toole 2000
Chapter 7 © Renée Danziger 2000
Chapter 8 © Malcolm Dando 2000
Chapter 9 © David Heymann 2000
Chapter 10 © Yves Beigbeder 2000
Chapter 11 © Donald A. Henderson 2000
Chapter 12 © William Foege 2000

All rights reserved. No reproduction, copy or transmission of this publication may be made
without written permission.

No paragraph of this publication may be reproduced, copied or transmitted save with written
permission or in accordance with the provisions of the Copyright, Designs and Patents Act
1988, or under the terms of any licence permitting limited copying issued by the Copyright
Licensing Agency, 90 Tottenham Court Road, London W1P 0LP.

Any person who does any unauthorised act in relation to this publication may be liable to
criminal prosecution and civil claims for damages.

The authors have asserted their rights to be identified as the authors of this work in accordance
with the Copyright, Designs and Patents Act 1988.

This book is printed on paper suitable for recycling and made from fully managed and sustained
forest sources.

10   9   8   7   6   5   4   3   2   1
09   08   07   06   05   04   03   02   01   00

Printed and bound in Great Britain by Antony Rowe Ltd, Chippenham, Wiltshire

Contents

Acknowledgements

An edited book depends on the support and goodwill of the contributors, and in this case, because I do not have a scientific or medical background, on an unseen network of scholars and practitioners who kindly suggested the most appropriate individuals or institutions to approach. It was a rewarding process, and I am grateful for the generosity of spirit shown to me by so many. Amongst the contributors, I am particularly grateful to Debarati Guha-Sapir for her early, enthusiastic support, which included a seemingly endless range of contacts.

My thanks to Publications Scientifiques, Institut Pasteur, for copyright consent to reprint the chapter by David Fidler, which first appeared in the *Bulletin of the Institute Pasteur*, 95 (1997), pp. 57–72.

Colonel John O'Shea, Director of the Strategic Outreach Program at the Strategic Studies Institute, US Army War College, was instrumental in securing a place for me at the Cantigny Conference 'Strategic Implications of Global Microbial Threats', 14 June 1996. I am indebted to the officers and staff of the Cantigny Foundation for a most interesting and worthwhile conference. Then and in subsequent communication, Professor Stephen Morse kindly furthered my rudimentary understanding of virology and bacteriology.

In Cambridge, Parmjot Bains, Rebecca Eldridge and Amanda Rees shared the findings of their own researches, which were a great help to me.

As always, Jack Shepherd, Jane Brooks, Angela Pollentine and Kathleen Shepherd provided the kind of support that arises from friendship as much as shared endeavour, something I will always prize.

Notes on the Contributors

Yves Beigbeder holds a doctorate in Public Law. A former WHO official, he is now an Adjunct Professor at Webster University, Geneva. He lectures on international organization and administration there and for UNITAR as a Senior Fellow. He has written several books and articles on UN organizations and their management, including WHO.

Manuel Carballo is the Coordinator of the International Centre for Migration and Health, Geneva.

Malcolm Dando is Professor of International Security at the School of Peace Studies, Bradford University. Trained as a zoologist, Professor Dando's current research interests include arms control and disarmament, biological and chemical weapons and global prohibition regimes.

Renée Danziger is a Lecturer in Health Policy at the London School of Hygiene and Tropical Medicine. She has been working on social and policy aspects of HIV/AIDS for the past ten years. During this time she has acted as a consultant for the New York City Human Rights Commission (AIDS Discrimination Unit) and the World Health Organization Global Programme on AIDS. She has also served as a member of the Technical Advisory Team of the Copenhagen-based Migration, Health and AIDS Project. Her other interests include the development of new conceptions of political power and powerlessness.

David P. Fidler obtained his JD from Harvard Law School and his BCL from the University of Oxford. He is currently Associate Professor of Law, Indiana University School of Law. He has written extensively on the international legal and political aspects of infectious diseases.

William H. Foege is an epidemiologist who is widely recognized as a key member of the successful campaign to eradicate smallpox in the 1970s. After serving as Chief of the CDC Smallpox Eradication Program, he was appointed Director of the US Centers for Disease Control in 1977. Dr Foege joined the Carter Center in 1986 as its Executive Director, Fellow for Health Policy and Executive Director of Global 2000. In 1992, he resigned as Executive Director of the Carter Center, but continues in his role as a Fellow and as Executive Director of the Task Force for Child Survival and Development.

Debarati Guha-Sapir is a Professor in the Department of Epidemiology, Faculty of Medicine, and the Centre for the Epidemiology of Disasters, University of Louvain.

Donald A. Henderson has served as Dean and Professor of Epidemiology and International Health at the Johns Hopkins School of Hygiene and Public Health since 1977. Prior to this, he served as Chief Medical Officer for the smallpox eradication programme of the World Health Organization in Geneva from 1966 to 1977.

David L. Heymann is the Director, Division of Emerging and other Communicable Diseases Surveillance and Control, at the World Health Organization. His distinguished career has also included extensive work on the Global Programme on AIDS, first as Chief of the Epidemiological Support and Research Unit and then as Chief of the Office of Research for four years. He has also published nearly one hundred scientific articles.

Kraig Klaudt directs the policy, strategy and promotion efforts of the World Health Organization's Global TB Programme in Geneva. Previously, he developed advocacy campaigns on international development, childhood nutrition and global militarization issues in the United States.

Jim Whitman is a Lecturer in the School of Peace Studies, Bradford University. He is the co-editor of the *Journal of Humanitarian Assistance* and general editor for the Macmillan Global Issues series.

Michael J. Toole is an epidemiologist with extensive field experience throughout the world, particularly in Africa and the Asia-Pacific region. As well as extensive periods as a medical director and adviser in Thailand and Somalia, he served in the International Health Program Office of CDC, responsible for providing and coordinating technical leadership to CDC's response to complex humanitarian disasters. He currently coordinates professional support for community health projects from the International Health Unit, Macfarlane Burnet Centre for Medical Research in Australia, with special emphasis on child survival and HIV/AIDS.

Abbreviations

ACT UP	AIDS Coalition to Unleash Power
APEC	Asia Pacific Economic Cooperation
APOC	African Programme for Onchocerciasis Control
ARI	Acute Respiratory Infection
AIDS	Acquired Immunodeficiency Syndrome
AZT	Zidovudine
BCG	Bacille Calmette-Guérin [TB vaccine]
BTWC	Biological and Toxin Weapons Convention
BW	Biological Weapons
CASU	Comité d'Action Sanitaire d'Urgence
CDC	Centers for Disease Control
CFR	Case Fatality Rate
CHW	Community Health Worker
CMR	Crude Mortality Rate
CNN	Cable News Network
COHRED	Council on Health Research for Development
COU	Concepts of Use
CRI	Community Research Initiative
CSM	Cerebro-Spinal Meningitis
CVI	Children's Vaccine Initiative
CW	Chemical Weapons
DANIDA	Danish International Development Assistance
DNA	Deoxyribonucleic Acid
DOTS	Directly Observed Treatment, Short-course
ECHO	European Community Humanitarian Office
ECJ	European Court of Justice
EID	Emerging infectious disease
EMC	Emerging and Other Communicable Diseases Surveillance and Control
ENHR	Essential National Health Research
EPI	Expanded Programme on Immunization [WHO]
EU	European Union
FAO	Food and Agriculture Organization
FDA	Food and Drug Administration
GATT	General Agreement on Tariffs and Trade
GPA	Global Programme on AIDS

HIV	Human Immunodeficiency Virus
ICMH	International Centre for Migration and Health
ICO	Intensified Cooperation with Countries
IDP	Internally Displaced Person
IEC	Information, Education and Communication
IHR	International Health Regulations
ILO	International Labour Organization
IUATLD	International Union Against TB and Lung Disease
KNCV	The Royal Netherlands Tuberculosis Association
MCH	Maternal and Child Health
MDR TB	Multidrug-Resistant Tuberculosis
MDT	Multidrug Therapy
MIRV	Multiple Independent Re-entry Vehicle
NAFTA	North American Free Trade Agreement
NGO	Non-Governmental Organization
NICD	National Institute of Communicable Diseases [India]
NIH	National Institutes of Health
OCP	Onchocerciasis Control Programme
PAHO	Pan-American Health Organization
PHARE	Poland, Hungary: Aid for Reconstruction of the Economy
PHLS	Public Health Laboratory Service
RNA	Ribonucleic Acid
RVF	Rift Valley Fever
SIDA	The Swedish official aid agency
TACIS	Technical Assistance for the Community of Independent States and Georgia
TB	Tuberculosis
UK	United Kingdom
UN	United Nations
UNDP	United Nations Development Programme
UNESCO	United Nations Educational, Scientific and Cultural Organization
UNFPA	United Nations Fund for Population Activities
UNHCR	United Nations High Commission for Refugees
UNICEF	United Nations Children's Fund
US	United States
VEE	Venezuelan Equine Encephalitis
WHO	World Health Organization
WMD	Weapons of Mass Destruction
WTO	World Trade Organization

1
Political Processes and Infectious Diseases

Jim Whitman

From the end of the Second World War, official pronouncement and public expectation in developed countries moved steadily toward the view that infectious disease was essentially conquered. There was a widely shared perception that although there remained large areas of the world still suffering the ravages of a variety of diseases, these could be met with the rapid pace of medical and scientific progress – or more directly, by the extension of existing mechanisms of control and cure. Postwar advances in material well-being and the attendant improvements in health and longevity, the introduction of penicillin and a range of vaccines, and a burgeoning faith in scientific and technological prowess gave this view a certain credence. In 1948, US Secretary of State George Marshall proclaimed that the conquest of all infectious diseases was imminent; in 1969, the US Surgeon-General William H. Stewart expressed his confidence that we had reached the frontiers in the field of contagious diseases.[1]

The number and variety of current infectious disease crises have engendered surprise, bewilderment and alarm that human disease agents have not been 'conquered'; that progress has not proved irreversible; that more of the same tactics for control of vectors or treatment of victims might not be sufficient to stem or reverse the tide; that the microbial world is more varied, numerous and adaptable than we had once supposed or hoped; and that the current and developing patterns of diseases worldwide are not only threats in themselves, but are also indices of a changed and changing balance between human and natural systems. In addition to the HIV/AIDS pandemic, we are experiencing global crises in malaria and TB, drug-resistant strains of bacteria once thought under control, the re-emergence of large-scale infectious disease in parts of the developed world – mumps and diphtheria in Russia, for example; the arrival of

1

familiar diseases in new areas (cholera in South America; yellow fever in Kenya); and the emergence of new, frighteningly lethal infectious viral diseases such as Ebola and Marburg.[2]

What now seems remarkable about those decades of confidence (and subsequent complacency) is not simply the emergence of diseases that have withstood years of concerted scientific research into aetiology and cure, nor even the resurgence of long-familiar diseases such as TB. More important is that behind the range of practical issues confronting us is a profound conceptual challenge, for it is now clear that Marshall's pronouncement was not so much wrong, or even premature, as *misconceived*.

This misconception does not turn on the scale and duration of scientific research and practical medicine required, but on a strangely curtailed notion of causal relations and a paradigmatic rather than 'web of life' view of biology. The relationship between the human and microbial worlds is of an order of complexity which defies a 'rolling back the frontiers' mentality, despite the persistence of martial metaphors in the nonscientific literature on disease. Whether or not a disease-free human future is a practical possibility – or indeed, even a logical one[3] – it is the argument of this chapter that our 'epidemic of epidemics' has political meaning which extends far beyond the immediate, often devastating human consequences of individual diseases and epidemics and our organizational responses. It is abundantly clear that disease surveillance, epidemiology, vector control or eradication and all manner of modern scientific, pharmaceutical and medical initiatives require varying degrees of political impetus for their initiation, maintenance or coordination. These necessities have not only intensified but have also undergone a change in character, as disease and the threat of disease have become a more global phenomenon, by way of extent, ease of transmission and possible repercussions.[4] But the political realm is much more closely and minutely bound up with natural systems than notions of 'stewardship' and 'management' of the environment might lead us to believe; and the quickening pace of their interactions is open to worsening possibilities in respect of disease, epidemic and pandemic.[5] The prospect is all the more sobering in a world in which millions continue to die from preventable and curable diseases and an apparent trajectory of scientific and medical progress has been met by the emergence of HIV/AIDS.

Infectious disease and the human condition

One need not subscribe to the view that infectious diseases are 'one of the fundamental parameters and determinants of human history'[6] to recognize the pivotal role they have played in many of the larger currents of human affairs and the often cruel progress of globalizing humanity.[7] From an apparently safe and medically advanced environment, it is tempting to regard epidemics and pandemics less as outcomes of powerful, complex and persistent dynamics and more as discrete, distant events – historically, part of the rhythm of the rise and fall of empires, but essentially 'acts of God', freaks of nature or vulnerabilities largely overcome by modernity. Yet a closer reading of history – of human expansion and migration,[8] of colonialism,[9] and early industrialization and urbanization[10] – begins to suggest a more continuous and less triumphant struggle.

The advancement of public health and scientific medicine are only a part of that struggle. At a more fundamental level, 'Like all other forms of life, humankind remains inextricably entangled in flows of matter and energy that result from eating and being eaten. However clever we have been in finding new niches in that system, the enveloping micro-parasitic-macroparasitic balances limiting human access to food and energy have not been abolished, and never will be.'[11] Depicting the human situation in this way is not asserting 'a new materialism in the form of an ecological vision of history in which disease plays a key role',[12] but siting humanity within planetary ecology, with its attendant dependencies, relationships and vulnerabilities. Seen in this way, the outbreak and spread of diseases are instances in the deep, complex and dynamic workings of pathogen–host relations, bacterial and viral traffic, the relationship between vectors and other species and the ability of the microbial world to mutate and adapt to changing conditions and new opportunities. As Lewis Thomas describes it, 'Disease usually represents the inconclusive negotiations for symbiosis . . . a biological misinterpretation of borders.'[13] The metaphor suggests not only particular cases of biological competition, but also the continuing evolution of life on Earth. Our comprehension of the living world appears highly tentative against the possibility that the number of bacteria might be above 1000 times the number currently recorded.[14]

Coevolution and a coexistence – adaptive, competitive, symbiotic and otherwise responsive to change – mark the human–microbial relationship. As Arno Karlen succinctly remarks, 'Infectious disease, then, is not nature's tantrum against humanity. Often it is an argument in what becomes a long marriage.'[15] This perspective does nothing to lessen present suffering or the historical import and human meaning of the diseases which have beset humanity across the millennia (and about which our knowledge is far from comprehensive), yet it does provide us with a context within which we can understand something of the predicament which is currently unfolding.

Growth, change, movement, expansion and adaptation are also the marks of mind and culture, and where the agency is social, arising from shared purpose and concerted effort, they are political, at least in the broadest sense. However much of this activity can be characterized as psychopathological is of no consequence to the adaptive capacities of disease agents unaffected by nobility or barbarism. War, colonial expansion and ecological devastation are as likely to engender reconfigurations in the relationship between the microbial and human worlds as are demographic shifts, changing patterns of land use or the ready access to remote regions of the world by many millions of human beings. The outline of the world's larger disease ecologies[16] can be discerned in the history of epidemics engendered by invasions, large migrations and the development of trade routes between distant lands.

Three broad conclusions can be drawn about infectious diseases and humanity on a planetary scale:

In microbial terms, globalization is already a reality. The influenza pandemic of 1918–19 which killed at least 21 million people was '. . . in terms of absolute numbers, the greatest single demographic shock that the human species has ever received. The Black Death and World Wars I and II killed higher percentages of the populations at risk, but took years to do so and were not universal in their destruction. The so-called Spanish Flu did most of its killing in a six-month period and reached almost every human population on Earth.'[17] Today, the speed and extent of worldwide commercial traffic and international tourism (which has grown at a rate of 7 per cent per year over four decades[18]) ensure global exchange still more rapid and pervasive. To this must be added what has been termed 'bio-invasions', engendered by the 'effective collapse of the world's ecological boundaries'[19] resulting in the movement of animal and plant species – including disease vectors such as the Asian tiger mosquito – into new ecosystems.

'Stability is a special case of change, not the natural order of things.'[20] Diseases and epidemics are not aberrations in the progress of scientific knowledge and technological prowess, but manifestations of life – of pathogens which 'have their own large role to play in shaping the diversity of living things on the earth'. Indeed, according to Christopher Wills, 'in order for us to preserve the diversity of a complex ecosystem like a rainforest or a coral reef, it will be necessary to preserve the pathogens as well as their hosts'.[21] Utopia is not a possibility and

passivity not an option; instead, we are offered a considerable challenge to our view of people and planet, perhaps beginning with the realization that environmental sustainability is a foundation of disease prevention. Even then, Joshua Lederberg offers us a humbling perspective:

At evolutionary equilibrium we would continue to share the planet with our internal and external parasites, paying some tribute, perhaps sometimes deriving from them some protection against more violent aggression. The terms of that equilibrium are unwelcome: present knowledge does not offer much hope that we can eradicate the competition. Meanwhile, our parasites and ourselves must share in the dues, payable in a currency of discomfort and precariousness of life. No theory lets us calculate the details; we can hardly be sure that such an equilibrium for earth even includes the human species even as we contrive to eliminate some of the others. Our propensity for technological sophistication harnessed to interspecies competition adds a further dimension of hazard.[22]

History may prove an inadequate guide: the possibilities are more extensive than recorded experience. Human activity has brought about environmental change not only on a large scale, but also on a systemic one. This is crucial to our understanding of the importance of global warming, ozone layer depletion and biodiversity loss: that their subsequent impacts on habitat viability, species resilience and distribution and the chemistry and physics of planetary life support all have direct, epidemiological implications.[23] Although it is not universally agreed that current trends in infectious disease will worsen disastrously,[24] it is plain that the avenues between local and global are broadening: infectious disease outbreaks can more easily become epidemics and epidemics become pandemics; at the same time, environmental disruption on a planetary scale can expose regions and populations to new disease risks, as is becoming clear with global warming.[25]

There are no grand historical narratives outside of the book of life: ecology does not punctuate human affairs but underlies them; and the larger currents of life affect and are affected by human activity. This is not a determinist position but a verifiable observation. As the biological foundations of the human condition increasingly become subject to the cumulative and synergistic repercussions of human activity, we can expect disruptions to the pattern of relationships between living things, some of which will take the form of infectious diseases, new and resurgent.

Political dynamics and infectious diseases

However, the occurrence of diseases and epidemics in human populations is not mere biology and chance. The social conditions of human beings are the largest determinants of their susceptibility to disease and these are politically shaped and driven. R. C. Lewontin makes an important distinction between the *agents* of diseases and their *causes*.[26] Distinguishing the tuberculosis bacilli as the agent of TB and poverty-induced malnutrition and depressed immunity as causes explains why only a fraction of the third of the human population which carry the bacilli actually manifest the disease. Likewise, while it is true that tropical areas provide the most favourable conditions for disease organisms,[27] the pattern and incidence of diseases in those areas and elsewhere – and morbidity and mortality statistics more generally – can be directly correlated to social conditions, a point amply demonstrated and acknowledged politically in Europe since at least the start of the nineteenth century.[28] Slum conditions including overcrowding, poor or non-existent sewerage, contaminated water, unregulated industrial pollution, uncontrolled proximity of vectors such as rats and mosquitoes, poor ventilation and little or no heating – the elements which comprised the lot of the poor during the industrialization of Europe – persist in the now-impoverished areas of the world, including the disenfranchised millions caught in the explosive urbanization of human populations now under way.[29]

The identification of political causation – say, the marginalization and impoverishment of peoples, whether the culprit is identified as an international institution or the incompetence or corruption of local officials – or the isolation of disease agents, easily brings us to a one-cause/one effect model of the incidence of infectious diseases, and of the relationship between human health and the environment more generally.[30] Lewotkin's distinction between agent and cause of disease is a valuable insight, but of little avail for predictive purposes – for determining the vulnerability of human populations against even well-known pathogens, particularly when environmental factors act as causal agents. More than thirty years ago, René Dubos observed: 'Disease presents itself simultaneously with so many different faces in any given area that it is usually impossible to attribute any one particular expression of it to one particular set of environmental circumstances.'[31] Of course, there are identifiable causal relations in epidemiology and appropriate responses in the political realm, stretching back to pre-scientific quarantine regimes.[32] The difficulty with the one-cause/one effect model is not only the complexity of human and environmental conditions which engender human–pathogen proximity and pathogen entry or adaptation, but also that the political forces which create and/ or sustain them are but rarely simple and linear, open to change by fiat.

It is clear, for example, that many of the water-borne diseases which kill millions every year do not pose a scientific or pharmaceutical challenge, most obviously in respect of infant deaths from diarrhoeal diseases. Depending on the nature of the prevailing conditions – lack of safe drinking water, inadequate sanitation, proximity to contaminated water and water-borne vectors, inadequate water for bathing and washing clothes – the nature and extent of illnesses and epidemics will vary considerably, within and between regions. The political dynamics driving these conditions are no less varied.

But so many of the environments in which human populations now find themselves – natural and political – greatly complicate both epidemiological assessments of risk and political responses. It is plain that the resurgence of diseases in the former Soviet Union, for example, is in part the outcome of its collapsed economy, chronic social dislocation and a grossly degraded natural environment,[33] but targeting disease agents rather than heightened vulnerabilities becomes ever less effective in such conditions, even as the political wherewithal to organize medical response shrinks still further. Aggregate economic prosperity and social stability are not in themselves good cause for complacency, however; in the United States, 'Age-adjusted mortality from infectious diseases increased 39 per cent [between 1980 and 1992].'[34]

There are few 'natural' environments anywhere in the sense that they have not been subject to some degree of human exploitation or intervention, with consequences for human health, both direct and indirect. For example, the attempts to eradicate or control disease vectors through the extensive use of pesticides result yearly in approximately one million cases of poisoning, with some 20 000 fatalities, principally in the developing world. Even in the United States, pesticides equivalent to four pounds weight for every man, woman and child are also applied.[35] It is far from clear what might be the legacy of extensive use of pesticides for the immune systems of those most affected,[36] but we are beginning to understand, belatedly, that 'insect and parasite resistance to biocides . . . contributed to the persistence and evolution of disease, especially in the tropical parts of the world. [. . .] Resistance emerged within a constellation of enormously complex social, medical, and ecological problems, many of which were poorly understood during the middle of the twentieth century. Among these problems, the limited knowledge of entomology, parasitology, and human immunology played a decisive role.'[37]

The microbial-environmental-human dynamics in many disease 'hot spots' are also politically volatile: war zones, refugee encampments and entire nations impoverished by a generation or more of violent conflict, to say nothing of the sites of continuing warfare which are more often than not in impoverished lands.[38] In addition to the obvious vulnerabilities inherent in these human predicaments, those enduring them are also highly susceptible to fluctuations in natural conditions – droughts, storms and floods – and through them, to the devastation of infrastructure and the spread or growth of disease vectors. Note the relations that typically characterize large-scale responses to 'humanitarian emergencies': a relatively secure and prosperous 'core', responding to an event on the periphery. Of course, an earthquake in Armenia is not equivalent to genocide in Rwanda, but both natural and anthropogenic humanitarian disasters share a number of interesting features: the disaster agents are often limited in duration, geographic extent and the degree to which they impinge on the interests of those distant and in some position to assist. All of these could be reversed in the case of an outbreak of a lethal and contagious disease. We are accustomed to the humanitarian interventions of military forces to protect and support beleaguered populations, but were those populations to pose a threat at the same time – were an afflicted community both victim and vector – the assumptions which underpin these operations would be shattered. Those who feel that such speculation falls outside the compass of Clauswitzian tenets would do well to recall that Clauswitz himself died as a result of cholera contracted on a military operation on the Prussian–Polish frontier.

A world in which infectious disease is a permanent risk is also shaped by local and regional conditions and initiatives, governmental and non-governmental. There cannot be said to be a global politics, but political initiatives of every kind can have reach and impact anywhere in the world. The way in which trade is organized and controlled, development conceived and funded, natural resources exploited and regulated – these and other fundamentals of human exchange are often subject to conditions and goals determined by powerful actors at some distance and mediated by local forces. To some degree, this also works in reverse – hence developed nations' efforts to stem the destruction of tropical rain forests. One of the more profound meanings of globalizing humanity is that we are coming to live within an encompassing political ecology, in which political acts and omissions have considerable direct and indirect effects, sometimes well beyond not only intent but also immediate comprehension, interacting with and sometimes compounded by the dynamics of the natural world – of which the spread of HIV/AIDS is the most obvious and compelling contemporary illustration. Although the origins and dissemination of HIV/AIDS is not known with certainty, it would appear that 'the virus has been present for many years in isolated groups in central Africa. Because outside contacts were minimal, the virus has rarely spread, and an epidemic could not be sustained. Once a sizeable reservoir of infection was established, however, HIV became pandemic.'[39] The agents of the disease – political, cultural, infrastructural, institutional – continue to interact and inform efforts to control it.[40]

The incidence of HIV/AIDS has not only opened up many social, cultural, biomedical and gender issues (at least in developed countries), but has also exposed previously unrecognized or under-examined issues ranging from social and health provision for marginalized groups to the politics of the international pharmaceutical industry.[41] The global and the local, the biological/medical and the political, all continue to create intricate sequences of action and reaction with respect to HIV/AIDS – as well as other diseases.

But even though consequences can be unforeseen and some political dynamics assume unwilled momentum, the initiating and responsive capacity of political agency – focused, committed and enduring – can still make considerable inroads into bettering the conditions of millions of people in the struggle to prevent, cure and sometimes eliminate infectious diseases. Hence the triumph of the eradication of smallpox (in 1977), of the progress made to reduce human suffering through global vaccination campaigns and the list of diseases for which some degree of international cooperation for eradication or control has been pledged.[42] The World Health Organization (and dedicated programmes within the wider UN system), the Centers for Disease Control in Atlanta and a host of other international, governmental and non-governmental organizations and foundations contribute to the struggle against disease, as well as to furthering surveillance efforts. Yet these institutions are not without conflicting political interests, nor are eradication programmes unencumbered with national-political, cultural, educational, or logistical difficulties and commercial interests.[43] And political willingness, at least as expressed in mission statements, must have secure financial and personnel underpinning, which is not always forthcoming. These deficiencies come at a time when public sector spending, including public health provision, is constrained even in the wealthiest parts of the world, while overseas development assistance continues to decline – a trend exacerbated by the demands of emergency humanitarianism.[44]

The dedication of epidemiologists, scientific researchers and health professionals can never be sufficient against the larger – and countervailing – forces which continue to entrench the gross deprivation of so much of humanity. Claims on justice aside, the fact that a quarter of humanity does not have access to safe drinking water and two thirds do not have adequate sanitation means that the health of all, rich and poor alike, is imperilled. This is more than just another rich world/poor world cleavage, because for infectious diseases there are no distant lands.

Yet old patterns of indifference, imperiousness and selfishness ascendant over humane decency persist, even in the face of a broadened but readily graspable conception of self-interest. AIDS vaccines have been tested on patients in Africa, Thailand and the Dominican Republic (with some having been given a placebo), for the treatment of patients in the developed world who can afford them.[45] And in the same year that 3000 children in Nigeria died in an outbreak of meningitis, an American company filed a patent application on the entire gene sequence of one of the meningitis bacteria, which 'could lead to royalties being paid on every treatment if a new vaccine against the illness is found'.[46]

Conclusion

Infectious diseases and the threat they pose may come to engage an ever greater part of the machinery of public policy, but epidemics which can be both swift and lethal are unlikely to inspire humane deliberation by publics or political authorities, as immigrant history in this century and the emergence of HIV/AIDS both demonstrate.[47] The practical challenges of coping with emerging and resurgent diseases are considerable, but perhaps the greater challenge is to recognize and comprehend the combination of forces driving them. The abstraction of politics from the dynamics of the living world is a conceit which cannot be sustained against a rapidly changing planetary ecology and a growing, globalizing human population. Infectious diseases are as much social phenomena as microbial ones and providing defence against them while bettering the lot of the millions currently afflicted is as much a political task as a medical and scientific one. The spur to this work is a reconception of the basis of human security. The persistence of disease agents is a constant reminder of the importance of that work; the possibility of a pandemic the price of failure.

Notes

1 George Marshall is cited in Laurie Garrett,*The Coming Plague: Newly Emerging Diseases in a World Out of Balance* (New York: Farrar, Straus & Giroux, 1994) p. 30; William Stewart is cited in Arno Karlen, *Plague's Progress: A Social History of Man and Disease* (London: Victor Gollancz, 1995) p. 3.

2 A comprehensive overview is provided by Kenneth F. Kiple (ed.), *The Cambridge History of Human Disease* (Cambridge: Cambridge University Press, 1993); accessible contemporary accounts include Garrett, ibid.; Anne E. Platt, 'Confronting Infectious Diseases,' in Lester R. Brown (ed.), *State of the World 1996* (London: Earthscan, 1996) pp. 114–32; and *The World Health Report 1996* (Geneva: World Health Organization, 1996).

3 'A more closely knit world . . . made it possible for illnesses such as plague and yellow fever, not normally diseases of humans, to seek out humans, with extraordinary lethality. Swelling populations provided a rapidly mutating swine influenza virus with hundreds of millions of hosts and tens of millions of victims in the early days of the twentieth century. Yet despite these numerous lessons from the past, those in the developed world have been led to believe that if only the new chronic diseases could be subdued, their world, at least, would become essentially disease-free. That this is even a state we should wish for ignored the millennia of symbiotic evolutionary adaptation of humans and pathogens.' Kenneth F. Kiple, 'The Ecology of Disease', in W. F. Bynum and Roy Porter (eds), *Companion Encyclopedia of the History of Medicine*, vol. 1 (London: Routledge, 1993) p. 377; see also William B. Schwartz, *Life Without Disease: the Pursuit of Medical Utopia* (Berkeley: University of California Press, 1997); Paul W. Ewald, *Evolution of Infectious Disease* (Oxford: Oxford University Press, 1994).

4 *The World Health Report 1996* (Geneva: WHO, 1996); Leon Gordenker, Roger A. Coate, Christer Jönsson and Peter Söderholm, *International Cooperation in Response to AIDS* (London: Pinter, 1995).

5 For an excellent overview, see A. J. McMichael, A. Haines, R. Slooff and S. Kovats (eds), *Climate Change and Human Health: an assessment prepared by a task group on behalf of the World Health Organisation, the World Meteorological Organisation and the United Nations Environment Programme* (Geneva: World Health Organization, 1996); A. J. McMichael, *Planetary Overload: Global Environmental Change and the Health of the Human Species* (Cambridge: Cambridge University Press, 1993).

6 William H. McNeill, *Plagues and Peoples* (London: Penguin, 1976) p. 268.

7 Ibid.; Hans Zinsser, *Rats, Lice and History* (New York: Bantam, 1965); Bernice A. Kaplan, 'Migration and Disease', in G. C. N. Mascie-Taylor and G. W. Lasker, *Biological Aspects of Human Migration* (Cambridge: Cambridge University Press, 1988) pp. 216–45; Alfred W. Crosby, *Ecological Imperialism: the Biological Expansion of Europe, 900–1900* (Cambridge: Cambridge University Press, 1986).

8 Crosby, ibid.; Philip D. Curtin, *Death By Migration: Europe's Encounter with the Tropical World in the Nineteenth Century* (Cambridge: Cambridge University Press, 1989).

9 Ibid.; Milton Lewis, *Disease, Medicine and Empire: Perspectives on Western Medicine and the Experiences of European Expansion* (London: Routledge, 1988).

10 John D. Post, *Food Shortage, Climatic Variability, and Epidemic Disease in Preindustrial Europe* (Ithaca: Cornell University Press, 1985).

11   William H. McNeill, *The Human Condition: an Ecological and Historical View* (Princeton: Princeton University Press, 1980) p. 74.

12   Charles E. Rosenberg, *Explaining Epidemics and Other Studies in the History of Medicine* (Cambridge: Cambridge University Press, 1982) p. 308.

13   Quoted in Ewald, op. cit., p. 3.

14   Edward O. Wilson, *The Diversity of Life* (London: Penguin, 1992) p. 143. Bacteria comprise only a fraction of microbial life. Viruses are also important disease agents and their coevolution with humanity is no less complex. See Ann Giudici Fettner, *The Science of Viruses* (New York: McGraw-Hill, 1990); Joshua Lederberg, 'Viruses and Humankind: Intercellular Symbiosis and Evolutionary Competition'; Stephen S. Morse, 'Examining the Origins of Emerging Viruses'; and Robert M. May, 'Ecology and Evolution in Host–Virus Associations', in Stephen S. Morse (ed.), *Emerging Viruses* (Oxford: Oxford University Press, 1993).

15   Karlen, op. cit., p. 16.

16   For a survey of the world's principal disease ecologies, see Kenneth F. Kiple (ed.), op. cit., pp. 447–543.

17   Alfred W. Crosby, 'Influenza,' in ibid., p. 810.

18   Henyk Handszuh and Sommerset R. Waters, 'Travel and Tourism Patterns', in Herbert L. DuPont and Robert Steffen (eds), *Textbook of Travel Medicine* (Ontario: B.C. Decker, 1997) pp. 20–6.

19   Chris Bright, *Life Out of Bounds: Bio-invasions in a Borderless World* (London: Earthscan, 1999).

20   A. W. DePorte, *Europe Between the Superpowers: The Enduring Balance* (New Haven: Yale University Press, 1986) p. xv.

21   Christopher Wills, *Plagues: Their Origin, History and Future* (London: Harper-Collins, 1996) pp. 290–1.

22   Joshua Lederberg, 'Medical Science, Infectious Disease, and the Unity of Mankind', *Journal of the American Medical Association*, vol. 260, no. 5 (1988) p. 685.

23   Thomas E. Lovejoy, 'Global Change and Epidemiology: Nasty Synergies', in Stephen S. Morse (ed.), op. cit., pp. 261–8; A. J. McMichael, A. Haines, R. Slooff and S. Kovats (eds), op. cit.

24   See Stephen Budiansky, 'Plague Fiction', *New Scientist*, vol. 148, no. 2006 (2 December 1995) pp. 28–33.

25   A. J. McMichael, A. Haines, R. Slooff and S. Kovats (eds), op. cit.

26   R. C. Lewontin, *The Doctrine of DNA: Biology as Ideology* (London: Penguin, 1993) p. 45.

27   Wills, op. cit., pp. 272–3; Kenneth F. Kiple (ed.), op. cit., pp. 447–543.

28   Dorothy Porter, 'Public Health', in W. F. Bynum and Roy Porter (eds), op. cit., pp. 1231–61; see also David Bradley, 'Health, Environment, and Tropical Development', in Bryan Cartledge (ed.), *Health and the Environment* (Oxford: Oxford University Press, 1994) pp. 127–49.

29   One reads the rationale behind much of the pre- and early Victorian public health reform with some dismay for its uncanny resemblances to the arguments of *laissez-faire* global capitalism: 'There was no role for the state or legislative reform in the view of the economist hygienists, for this would undermine individual freedom and initiative. [. . .] They sought instead a programme of amelioration through religious indoctrination of the poor into the ways of moral behaviour. Their answer to the claim that civilization

produced the ills of society, such as poverty, was simply to say that the poor were as yet uncivilized. Their answer to the question, "what was the cause of poverty?" was the poor themselves and who, once they were educated into the ways of civilized behaviour, would eliminate it.' Ibid., p. 1240.

30 The phrase 'one-cause/one effect model' appears in Ross Hume Hall, *Health and the Global Environment* (Cambridge, Polity Press, 1990).

31 René Dubos, from *Man, Medicine and Environment*, quoted in Kenneth F. Kiple (ed.) p. 474.

32 Oleg P. Schepin and Waldemar V. Yermakov, *International Quarantine* (Madison, Conn.: International Universities Press, 1991).

33 Murray Feisbach and Alfred Friendly Jr., *Ecocide in the USSR: Health and Nature under Siege* (London: Aurum Press, 1992).

34 Robert B. Pinner, et al., 'Trends in Infectious Diseases Mortality in the United States', *Journal of the American Medical Association*, vol. 275 (1996) pp. 189–93.

35 Mark L. Winston, *Nature Wars: People vs. Pests* (Cambridge: Harvard University Press, 1997) pp. 11–12.

36 See John Wargo, *Our Children's Toxic Legacy: How Science and Law Fail to Protect Us from Pesticides* (New Haven: Yale University Press, 1996).

37 Ibid., p. 62. 'Furthermore, enormous amounts of medical antimicrobials are used for the production of animal food around the world ... More than half the total production of all antimicrobials is used in farm animals, either for disease prevention or for growth promotion. Drug-resistant bacteria are passed through the food chain to the consumer, where they may cause disease or transfer the resistance to human pathogens.' World Health Organization, op. cit., p. 19.

38 For example, see Saul Bloom, John M. Miller, James Warner and Philippa Winkler, *Hidden Casualties: Environmental, Health and Political Consequences of the Persian Gulf War* (London: Earthscan, 1994); see also *Medicine and War*, 'A quarterly journal of international medical concerns on war and other social violence.'

39 Alan M. Brandt, 'Acquired Immune deficiency Syndrome (AIDS)', in Kenneth F. Kiple (ed.), op. cit., p. 549.

40 See Jonathan Mann and Daniel Tarantola (eds), *AIDS in the World II* (Oxford: Oxford University Press, 1996).

41 See for example, Cindy Patton, *Last Served? Gendering the HIV Pandemic* (London: Taylor & Francis, 1994); Ruth Faden, Gail Geller and Madison Powers (eds), *AIDS, Women and the Next Generation: Towards a Morally Acceptable Public Policy for HIV Testing of Pregnant Women and Newborns* (Oxford: Oxford University Press, 1991); Julia Epstein, *Altered Conditions: Disease, Medicine and Storytelling* (London: Routledge, 1995); Tim Rhodes and Richard Hartnoll, *AIDS, Drugs and Prevention: Perspectives on Individual and Community Action* (London: Routledge, 1996); Lynn R. Brown, *The Potential Impact of AIDS on Population and Economic Growth Rates*, Agriculture and the Environment Discussion Paper 15 (Washington, DC: International Food Policy Research Institute, 1996); Steven Epstein, *Impure Science: AIDS, Activism, and the Politics of Knowledge* (Berkeley: University of California Press, 1996).

42 See 'Recommendations of the International Task Force for Disease Eradication', *Morbidity and Mortality Weekly Report*, vol. 42 (Atlanta: Centers for Disease Control, 31 December 1993).

43 Javed Siddiqi, *World Health and World Politics: the World Health Organization and the UN System* (London: Hurst, 1995); Paul F. Basch, *Vaccines and World Health: Science, Policy and Practice* (Oxford: Oxford University Press, 1994); Leon Gordenker, Roger A. Coate, Christer Jönsson and Peter Söderholm, op. cit.

44 Judith Randel and Tony German (eds), *The Reality of Aid, 1997–1998: an Independent View of Development Cooperation* (London: Earthscan, 1998).

45 Lucy Johnston and Ruaridh Nicol, 'AIDS Drugs Cut to "Guinea Pigs"' and 'AIDS, Africans and the Side-effects of Poverty', *London Observer*, 8 June 1997 (Editorial).

46 David King and Paul Brown, 'Firm Attempts to Patent Meningitis Bacteria', *The Guardian*, 7 May 1998.

47 'The double helix of health and fear that accompanies immigration continues to mutate, producing malignancies on the culture, neither fatal nor easily eradicated.' Alan M. Kraut, *Silent Travelers: Germs, Disease and the 'Immigrant Menace'* (Baltimore: The Johns Hopkins University Press, 1994) p. 272; see also Randy Shilts, *And the Band Played On: Politics, People and the AIDS Epidemic* (New York: St. Martin's Press, 1987).

2
Poverty, Development, Population Movements and Health

Manuel Carballo

> The world has suddenly become unusually complex and far less intelligible. The old order has collapsed, but no one has yet created a new one.
>
> Vaclav Havel, President of the Czech Republic

Introduction

The twentieth century has seen some of the most dramatic political, economic and technological changes that have ever taken place, and the numbers of people directly or indirectly affected by them have been greater than at any other time in recent history. In many ways the world has become smaller and more homogenized.

Faster, more efficient and cheaper communications systems have done much to create more universally shared value systems and patterns of behaviour than at any time in history. Throughout the world there have also been major changes in patterns of governance, and in general there has been a gradual but measurable trend away from top-down, authoritarian government structures towards more representative and participatory government. More people are living in pluralistic political systems than ever before, and the number of democratically elected governments has increased dramatically over the past twenty years or so.[1]

Patterns of international cooperation have also changed, and throughout much of the developed and less developed world new political and economic alliances have been forged on a scale rarely seen outside the context of colonial administrations. Pushed by the growing pressure of a global economic system and by an apparent increasing desire for broader international defence agreements, the relationship between many countries and regions has become closer and more symbiotic than ever.

Economic growth, if measured simply in terms of aggregate global incomes, has accelerated and become a core feature of the latter part of the twentieth century. Meanwhile, the impact of a technology-driven change is being felt everywhere, and more people are now moving away from agricultural subsistence economies to quasi-industrial and post-industrial social systems and ways of life.

To what extent the benefits normally accruing from these changes are, or will in the future be shared equitably nevertheless remains debatable. The evidence to date suggests that their distribution has by no means been a fair one. Economic disparities between richer and poor countries have widened, and even within many individual countries, the gap between rich and poor people has become more apparent. The income differential between the richest and poorest fifth of the world's population has more than doubled in the space of 30 years, and over 1 billion people are estimated to be living in absolute poverty according to World Bank criteria.

Nor have patterns of economic development been linear, and there have been dramatic instances of marked deterioration in economic indicators in countries that were previously considered industrialized and with well-established economies. Thus, while the most apparent gap has been between African countries and the rest of the world, major differences have also emerged between west and east European countries. At a global level, and in less well developed regions of the world, over eighty countries now have lower per capita incomes than they did fifteen years ago.

Highly visible improvements, including the apparent growth in per capita GNP, the share of households with clean water (up by 50 per cent), the proportion of households with access to electricity, and food productivity, have thus masked major and growing pockets of absolute as well as relative poverty. More than 2 billion people still do not have electricity; 1.7 billion have no sewage disposal; and 1 billion do not have access to clean drinking water. The World Bank estimates that these conditions contribute directly to 2–3 million infant and child deaths per year.[2]

In many countries the introduction of so-called participatory and representative government has not been supported by equivalent improvements in education, and achieving global literacy remains an obstinate challenge throughout the world. In some regions moreover, there has been an evident growth in nationalism, more frequent and vociferous expressions of ethnic identity, and a greater commitment to maintaining or assuming power of so-called historical rights to scarce water and land.

The benefits of technological growth have also been highly skewed both in terms of regions and economic systems. In many parts of the world, the growth in technology has outpaced the capacity of some countries to generate and implement the social policies required to accommodate that growth without causing major social disruption. And while much of the population movement taking place everywhere clearly reflects widening visions of the world, and an improved capacity to move, many of the reasons behind much of the mass movement are the same economic, territorial, and political and ethnic-religious inequities of old.

Thus, at the end of the twentieth century, development and its impact on quality of life and health has been a highly variable phenomenon. At best, the evident benefits of development have been poorly distributed. At worst, much of the development that is taking place is in danger of bypassing many people. The reasons are no doubt legion and complex. In this chapter some of those reasons are explored.

Development projects and displacement

No century was more associated with the concept and possibility of societal engineering than the twentieth. The capacity to alter the environment has been enormously enhanced and the possibility of envisaging new, man-made ecological and production systems has grown with it. Internationally financed development projects to construct dams, irrigation schemes, hydroelectric power plants, new waterways and roads have become more common everywhere, and have gone far in altering the economic viability and capacity of countries. The overall social and health cost of many of these schemes have nevertheless been high and in many instances they have prompted new types of poverty and disenfranchised millions of people.

The forced displacement of people in order to accommodate or adjust to major engineering schemes has become virtually synonymous with contemporary development. Especially, but by no means only in developing countries, internationally financed construction projects involving major dams (as many as 300 per year) and other infrastructure schemes (roads and waterways) are estimated to be displacing as many as 10 million people per year. Over the past 12 years or so, their impact has been to uproot and forcibly displace between 80 and 90 million people.[3]

All too little attention has been given to the impact this is having on the lives of the communities and individuals concerned or to the need for resettlement programmes. For example, until recently, economic and social development investment intended to enhance the options of the people displaced by these schemes has rarely been an integral part of development plans. Instead there has been an implicit tendency for displacement to be seen as an unfortunate but necessary ancillary of development schemes and for resettlement to be viewed as the responsibility of those who are displaced.

The impact of development schemes has been various, but in general their capacity to disrupt societies, disorganize local economic structures, and adversely affect the lives of people and communities may have been grossly underestimated. By their very design, development schemes produce complex and far-reaching changes in ecology, availability and distribution of natural resources. They also inevitably touch many aspects of social life, and the history of these schemes is replete with examples of forced displacement that has in turn distorted traditional cultures and value systems, and eroded local community networks and social support systems. Their impact on local economy and productivity, no matter how rudimentary, can and has been equally negative. At worst, forcing the displacement of communities has meant the dispersion of families, directing individuals into new and often socially inhospitable environments. These have sometimes been able to offer few opportunities for people with limited education and training, or provide the financial base needed for them to invest in resolving needs.

Individual material losses have often compounded family and societal disorganization, and made the people caught by displacement all the more vulnerable. There is growing evidence that displacement in the wake of development and major engineering projects that have been designed to improve overall quality of life have actually increased rather than decreased poverty. Dismantling of local production systems – no matter how simple – can be difficult if not impossible for poorly educated unskilled people to adjust to, and it is exactly these types of people who have been primarily affected by these schemes. Balancing losses and preventing impoverishment through new income generation and distribution have been neither easy nor especially successful. More importantly, trying to do so has not even been systematically built into the design of such schemes.

One of the more obvious impacts of development schemes has been the expropriation or reduced access to land. As a result, imposed landlessness has often followed in the path of development schemes, and with it has gone the mainstay of family economies which, even though imperfect, nevertheless provided bases that are difficult to replace. Loss of land that has often been passed down through generations of families and constituted the mainstay of family economies has effectively reduced the possibility of self-sufficiency and often broken the special bond that exists between agricultural people and their land.[4] As well as creating chronic food deficiency,[5] it has forced many people, especially those with limited education and skills into new social and economic situations that are difficult to navigate and cope with.

New and often more pernicious forms of poverty have emerged[6] and to date few ways of adequately compensating families have emerged. In part this is because the close ties that exist between agricultural people and their land are complex and difficult to assess and quantify. Certainly they are difficult to substitute for. Breaking with the land they have worked and depended on often means a radical departure from an entire worldview, from the cultures and ways of dealing with life that have evolved with them.[7]

What can be more easily determined and quantified are the more obvious losses that have occurred in terms of amount of land and livestock lost. In Kenya, for example, the impact of one hydroelectric power scheme was to limit the land holdings of resettled people from 13 to 6 hectares and reduce their livestock by over a third.[8] The World Bank has reported equally adverse outcomes in Indonesia and Brazil, and there are no doubt others.

For many people, forced displacement means the onset of joblessness and, in the absence of skills training and special programmes to prepare them for new occupations, chronic unemployment can and does quickly follow. Even in the presence of job training and the eventual development of saleable skills, the reality is that economic opportunities for people forcibly moved from one location to another are constrained by the poverty and limited economic development of the places they move to. Where jobs are scarce for everyone, there are few incentives to providing preferential employment for resettled people, and even where there is no preferential treatment of resettled people, they are nevertheless often seen as economic threats or liabilities.

Reports from both developed and developing countries, urban as well as rural areas, indicate that joblessness is high among people who are displaced by development schemes.[9] Creating jobs for them is meanwhile seen as costly and socially difficult. Even when job creation programmes have been set up, the sustainability of the jobs that have been created has not been demonstrated. In general, however, creating jobs has rarely been given high priority by national authorities or international agencies. All too often the result has been social and economic exclusion within the communities they are moved to and a further distancing from the possibility of re-establishing their lives.

Homelessness is another recurrent consequence of forced disruption in the context of large development schemes.[10] Just as with land and employment, the opportunities for displaced people to find, rent or purchase homes are limited. Building new homes can mean little more than temporary shanty housing in squatter settlements, or on land of precarious tenure that is prone to confiscation by local authorities.[11] Evidence suggests that few resettlement schemes have been able to facilitate the necessary access to new building land, nor have they been able to allocate the financial support required to provide better quality housing. A World Bank report[12] on a resettlement programme in Cameroon-Duala found that of over 2000 families who had been displaced, less than 5 per cent received loans to offset the cost of land. This is not an unusual outcome: in China almost 20 per cent of people relocated as part of a reservoir construction (not financed by the World Bank) soon became homeless and destitute.

The health consequences further compound the impact of development schemes. Poverty, unemployment and homelessness, for example, are often additionally impacted by ecological factors exposing people to new vectors and risk situations. The Nam Pong dam in Thailand provoked marked increases in local rates of river fluke and hookworm morbidity as a result of the poor waste disposal and poor living conditions that people were moved to. The incidence and prevalence of malaria also increased. Similarly, around the Akossombo dam in Ghana, the prevalence of schistosomiasis rose from 1.8 per cent to 75 per cent as a direct result of the ecological changes brought about by construction of the dam.[13] And an irrigation project in Mauritania produced rates of Rift Valley Fever (RVF) that far exceeded even the expectations of planners who had anticipated some increase.[14] The water pollution that was created in the region also provoked frequent and severe gastrointestinal disease epidemics.[15]

Political conflict and displacement

Forced displacement of people has taken other forms too, and conflict has been a prime cause of uprooting. While war in one form or another has been endemic to most periods of history, the twentieth century saw national and international conflict taken to new levels of intensity and scope. Although many of the more recent conflicts have been relatively small in historical terms, their impact on population displacement has accelerated.

Since 1980 an estimated 130 conflicts have erupted around the world[16] and in 1980 alone it is estimated that over 100 million people were directly affected by them. By 1991 that figure had risen to over 310 million. Between 1990 and 1995 at least 70 states were involved in 93 wars that resulted in the deaths of more than 6 million people, and the uprooting of approximately 70 million people from their homes, communities and countries.[17]

The changing nature of conflict, and its focus on or around the purposeful disruption of civil society has given rise to a new term, 'complex emergency'. Recent conflicts have targeted civilian populations, seeking to cause high civilian casualties, and setting out to destabilize civil society and governance. They have become increasingly and more visibly associated with human rights abuses, the systematic rape of women, girls and in many cases men for purposes of humiliation and as instruments of ethnic cleansing. Ethnic cleansing has in general become a more frequent characteristic of intra- and inter-country conflicts, and in many recent complex emergencies has involved the ritualistic razing of religious and administrative buildings, hospitals and schools.

Although there has inevitably been considerable variation between countries and conflicts, a large proportion of the wars that have occurred over the past twenty years have involved poor countries with frail national infrastructures. One of the immediate implications of this has been the further weakening of the capacity of countries to meet the basic needs of people, and conditions have been created in which previous health gains have been rapidly negated. Opportunities for post-conflict reconstruction and development have also been additionally constrained[18] and for many of the countries concerned, the incapacity to rebound after debilitating conflicts has led to renewed instability and fighting.

Thus while it is true that at a global level there has been a generalized movement toward pluralistic society and more democratic government, around the world there have also been major denials of equity and citizenship with serious implications for poverty, development and health. Conservative estimates of the number of people killed in the last 8–10 years of conflict are 6 million. Millions more have been severely injured and disabled, effectively placing them outside the parameters of development potential. So extensive has been the 'indiscriminate' use of landmines that even in times of post-conflict peace, 2500 people are estimated to be injured through anti-personnel mines each month, one every 20 minutes.[19] This type of use of land mines in civilian areas has not only increased the risk of serious injury and death, but it has made the resettlement of mined areas impossible, thus making social and economic reconstruction precarious if not impossible.

Table 2.1   People of concern to UNHCR

Refugee receiving countries	Number	Refugee receiving countries	Number
AFRICA		Hong Kong	6,875
Algeria	190,267	India	233,370
Angola	9,381	Iran	2,030,359
Benin	5,960	Iraq	112,957
Burkina Faso	28,381	Kazakstan	15,577
Côte d'Ivoire	327,696	Kyrgyzstan	16,707
Cameroon	46,407	Nepal	126,815
Central African	36,564	Pakistan	1,202,703
Republic		Saudi Arabia	9,852
Congo	20,451	Syria	27,759
D. R. Congo (ex-Zaire)	675,973	Thailand	107,962
Djibouti	25,076	Turkey	8,166
Egypt	6,035	Turkmenistan	15,580
Ethiopia	390,528	Vietnam	34,400
Gambia	6,924	Yemen	53,546
Ghana	35,617	Asia: other countries	14,479
Guinea	63,854		
Guinea-Bissau	15,401	*Total Asia*	4,808,624
Kenya	223,640		
Liberia	120,061	*EUROPE*	
Libya	7,747	Austria	29,745
Mali	18,234	Belarus	30,525
Mauritania	15,880	Belgium	36,060
Niger	25,845	Croatia	165,395
Nigeria	8,486	Denmark	53,302
Rwanda	25,257	Finland	10,248
Senegal	65,044	Macedonia (FYR)	5,089
Sierra Leone	13,532	France	151,329
South Africa	22,645	Germany	1,266,000
Sudan	393,874	Greece	5,780
Tanzania	498,732	Hungary	7,537
Togo	12,589	Italy	71,630
Uganda	264,294	Netherlands	103,425
Zambia	131,139	Norway	57,000
Africa: other countries	9,966	Russian Federation	205,458
		Slovenia	10,014
Total Africa	3,741,480	Spain	5,685
		Sweden	191,200
ASIA		Switzerland	84,413
Afghanistan	18,775	United Kingdom	96,905
Armenia	218,950	Yugoslavia (FR)	563,215
Azerbaijan	233,000	Europe: other countries	16,084
Bangladesh	30,692		
China	290,100	*Total Europe*	3,166,039

LATIN AMERICA		USA	596,900
Argentina	10,430	*Total North America*	720,119
Belize	8,534		
Costa Rica	23,176	OCEANIA	
Mexico	34,569	Australia	59,029
Latin America: other	11,721	Papua New Guinea	10,176
countries		Oceania: other	5,749
Total Latin America	88,430	countries	
		Total Oceania	74,954
NORTH AMERICA			
Canada	123,219		

Source: UNHCR, 1997

The denial of food and access to water and medical supplies as a weapon of war has been widespread, and has created conditions of famine and food shortage. The impact of this has been felt long after conflicts have come to an end. In Angola, one of the richest natural resource countries of Africa, 940 000 people remain in desperate need of food aid; and malnutrition in under-five year old children has become virtually the norm even during the current 'post-conflict' period.[20]

How many people have been forced to move by recent complex emergencies is difficult to estimate. One of the most serious implications of recent wars for social and health development has been the massive displacement of people they have precipitated. Over the course of the past ten years, at least 70 million people, that is to say more than the combined populations of Belgium, Denmark, Finland, Greece, Ireland, Luxembourg, Norway, Portugal, Sweden, and Switzerland have been forced to move from their homes, their towns and villages, and from their countries. At different times over the past ten years, refugees and internally displaced people have been spread over 100 countries, not only suffering themselves, but also placing new and additional loads on receiving communities and countries.

While the number of displaced people has come down significantly between 1997 and 1999, this has been a result of 'repatriation' programmes promoted by third party countries rather than a voluntary and spontaneous return. Nor has repatriation always or necessarily been indicative of cessation of conflict and the re-establishment of security. Indeed, the resettlement of IDPs and refugees in many countries and in their communities of origin is a fragile process and in itself is seriously affecting the potential for socio-economic development.

To what extent the displacement of people in complex emergencies leads to chronic social disorganization and personal dysfunction varies according to many factors. One is the highly sex- and age-selective nature of displacement in conflict settings. In general, and unless there is time for careful evacuations to be planned and carried out, the very young and the old are limited in their capacity to move easily and freely. Mortality in both groups is high when they do move, and in many situations older people simply choose to be left behind. For a variety of reasons men and boys of military age are also soon lost to their families, targeted by hostile forces, recruited into national armies, or fleeing the prospect of both. Few get the chance to leave with their families. The intentional disruption and disorganization of families and lifestyles seriously affects the coping capacity of people and impairs the ability of survivors to adapt both during conflicts and after they come to an end.[21]

Homes and communities of origin often remain in contested or heavily mined areas, making any return unlikely and the implications for health and economic development poor. The long duration of recent conflicts has also meant that displacement itself is tending to be of longer duration too. As a result, refugee camps are taking on a different character and role and the risk of increasing dependency on humanitarian aid has been heightened while the capacity of refugees and displaced people to assume responsibility for themselves has decreased. In general, however, the impact of conflict and displacement on physical and mental health is to create conditions that in many ways mimic those of poverty and under-development, with all the attendant health characteristics of poverty. The positive role of camps in securing stable health conditions can meanwhile take weeks if not months to emerge. During July and August 1992, daily crude mortality rates among Mozambican refugees in Chambuta camp who had been there for less than one month were reported to be 8 per 10000. This was four times the death rate of refugees who had been in the camp between one and three months, which was itself 16 times higher than for non-displaced populations in Mozambique.[22] Similarly, among Rwandan refugees fleeing into the northern Kivu region of Eastern Zaire in 1994, crude daily mortality rates reached between 25 and 50 per 10000 people per day.

Although refugee camps tend to stabilize health conditions, especially in comparison to what transpires during the acute phase, this is not always the case. Among Somali refugees in Ethiopia in 1988 the crude mortality rate and under-five-year mortality rates actually increased and remained high for almost 18 months after the initial influx. Approximately 75 per cent of the displaced children under five years died within a six-month period of uprooting, and the proportion of children under five in the overall displaced population fell from 18.3 per cent to 7.8 per cent.[23] In Bosnia, crude mortality rates reported in Muslim enclaves during the height of the war in 1993 were approximately four times pre-war rates, and up to 1996 the health of displaced people remained inferior to that of the population as a whole.[24]

It is the youngest infants, however, who are at the greatest risk. In Sarajevo, perinatal mortality rates rose from approximately 15 per 1000 live births prior to the war, to 39 per 1000 during it. Most deaths were due to conditions such as respiratory distress and asphyxia, which would have presented few problems under other circumstances. In the artificially impoverished conditions of the war, however, where 12 000 health personnel were lost and where 75 per cent of all hospital equipment was destroyed, problems of this kind soon came to be life threatening. The frequency of congenital abnormalities also tripled, and while it was difficult to pinpoint any single factor, the lack of folic acid in food supplementation for pregnant women may have played a role. The number of low-birth-weight babies also rose from a pre-war rate of 5.3 to 12.8 for almost the entire five years of the conflict.[25]

The vulnerability of under-five year old children in general is classic and related to a number of factors, not least of which is the incapacity of families to remain intact and provide the care and support that children require. Unaccompanied children become a major risk group. Among Rwandan refugees in north Kivu where there were more than 10 000 such children and where most were orphans, daily death rates during the first six weeks were 20 to 80 times higher than Rwandan estimates for under-five mortality before the crisis.[26]

The causes of high mortality vary, but poverty-mimicking factors predominate. Food shortages are a common factor. Among displaced people in Sarajevo, weight losses of up to 12 kilos were common during the 1992–3 period, and even two years after the Dayton Agreement, the number of people in Sarajevo still dependent on humanitarian food rations is estimated to be at least 30 000. Acute protein-energy malnutrition is widespread in conflict situations and quickly leads to heightened mortality, especially from communicable diseases. The deficiencies in shelter, clean water and food that characterize much of refugee camp life quickly contribute to other problems, and cholera epidemics are not unusual.[27] In the Goma camps of eastern Zaire more than 90 per cent of the estimated 50 000 deaths that occurred in the first month of refuge were caused by watery or bloody diarrhoea.[28] Cholera epidemics were reported among refugees in Malawi, Zimbabwe, Swaziland, Nepal, Bangladesh, Turkey, Afghanistan, Burundi and Zaire and in Goma. In eastern Zaire, a cholera outbreak occurred within the first week of the arrival of refugees, and over 90 per cent of deaths in the first month were attributed to diarrhoeal disease.[29] Cholera case fatality rates in refugee camps often reached 30 per cent.

Breakdowns in health care services and health promotion are a common feature of all complex emergencies, and can be more important causes of mortality than war injuries. Among the first of services to be affected by emergencies are those providing immunization. Problems of procurement and storage of vaccines, breakdowns in the cold chain, incapacity of health care workers to travel and out-reach to populations, as well as the high mobility of target populations, make it difficult to provide vaccination. Measles is one of the most immediate and dangerous problems in these situations. In one eastern Sudan refuge camp the measles-specific death rate among children under five years of age was 30 per 1000 per month and the case fatality rate (CFR), based on reported cases, reached almost 30 per cent.[30] Similarly high measles death rates have been reported in other complex emergencies in Somalia, Bangladesh, and Ethiopia.[31]

In Bosnia, where immunization coverage prior to the war was very high (coverage for TB, poliomyelitis, measles, diphtheria, pertussis, tetanus in 1991, was 81 per cent, 81 per cent, 76 per cent, and 79 per cent respectively), an International Centre for Migration and Health (ICMH) survey in 1996 indicated that immunization coverage fell dramatically among internally displaced people. In the case of measles, for example, mothers' reports indicated that it fell to less than 37 per cent among displaced children aged 0–4, and to 66 per cent among 5–9 year olds. Based on available vaccination cards, it was slightly less than 24 per cent in children aged 0–4 years, and 43 per cent in children aged 5–9 years.

The exposure of refugees to new diseases is also a problem if people are being moved from low disease endemic areas to areas of high endemicity. Thus, for example, refugees who moved from Cambodia to Thailand in 1979, highland Ethiopians who fled to eastern Sudan in 1985, and highland Rwandans who went to Zaire in 1994, all became more exposed to malaria and experienced elevated rates of the disease.[32] Opportunities for protecting refugees against these diseases are often poor, and humanitarian organizations and others may simply not take the problem into account, not realizing the nature of the problem and also assuming that there is a natural immunity in the group. In most crises, the danger of acute respiratory infections is also common. The overcrowding, poor ventilation, and lack of heating that is common to many emergency situations, as well as the normal vulnerability of young children, make acute respiratory infections an especially common and dangerous problem. In Bosnia acute respiratory infection became a frequent cause of complications in young infants, and one of the main causes of perinatal and neonatal mortality.[33] In Thailand, Somalia, Sudan, Honduras and Malawi acute respiratory infections have been cited as one of the three main causes of mortality in refugee camps, particularly among children.[34] Many of the health problems resulting from forced complex emergency displacement persist long after the emergencies have passed. There are many reasons for this, but one of the more critical is the policy and logistical gap between relief and development work. Humanitarian agencies may have as their specific mandate the provision of relief during the emergency, and may well be specialized in doing just that. Once emergencies – however defined are over, these agencies may feel compelled to leave. The assumption is that once the violence has subsided and the high levels of disease-related mortality have subsided, the danger has passed. In fact the transition from relief to development and reconstruction presents almost as many hazards and concerns as the emergency phase. And continued investment in refugees may also be politically undesirable for fear of helping them 'settle' where they are.

Attempts to encourage refugees and IDPs to return to their countries of origin are meanwhile often encouraged by decreasing the help provided to them in camps. At the same time there may be inadequate investment in the communities that they are expected to return to, and if and when they do return to them they are again faced with many of the same health problems they experienced during flight. The return of refugees from other countries in Europe to areas of Bosnia that have not been rehabilitated in terms of health care and social services, for example, will be fraught with new difficulties and problems. To what extent the lack of services in a country where 75 per cent of all hospital and clinic equipment was destroyed and where 12 000 health care staff were lost[35] could go on to create instability and further mobility, remains to be seen. The high loss of heads of household and persisting problems with trauma, may further impede the capacity of people returning to devastated regions to participate in a process of social reconstruction.

Urbanization

Of all the social changes that took place throughout the world in the twentieth century, and particularly in developing countries, none was more dramatic or far-reaching for public health than the rapid growth of urban centres. Throughout much of the 1960s and 70s the process of urbanization was largely seen as a positive indicator of development. It was felt to be demonstrative of the economic growth of countries and the capacity of cities to industrialize and absorb a new labour force drawn from rural areas. The concentration of populations in and around urban centres was also felt to be one of the factors that would facilitate the provision of health, education and other social services.

For a variety of reasons many of these assumptions have not been borne out. In poorer countries, the continued exodus of people from rural to urban areas, and the natural growth within new urban centres, has placed demands on emerging cities that are difficult if not impossible to meet. Between 1980 and 1985 urban growth reached a peak of 4.6 per cent for developing countries, and by 1990 urban growth for the world in general reached 3.1 per cent.[36] In developing countries, where the resources of cities are least capable of meeting the needs of newcomers, the rate of growth was 4.5 per cent in 1990. By 1990, 2400 million people, that is to say 45 per cent of the population of the world, were living in urban areas, and it is now anticipated that within the next several years, more than 50 per cent of the world's population will be living in urbanized areas. Between 1990 and 2025 it is projected to increase threefold.[37]

In countries experiencing economic crises, further cuts in already inadequate social and infrastructural investment can seriously impair water supply, sanitation, and health care. Per capita expenditures on health in developing countries which were already exceptionally low at the beginning of the 1980s (average of US$ 4 per person per year in 92 developing countries compared with an average of 220 dollars per person per year in 32 more affluent countries)[38] have continued to fall. With it, the capacity of urban centres to cope with growing population loads (natural and migration-related) has also decreased over time. Between 1970 and 1985 the size of the urban population living in absolute poverty increased by 73 per cent, from 177 million to 306 million, while the increase within rural populations was 11 per cent.[39]

Squatter settlements and peri-urban slums now typify much of the urban scene of developing countries, and as much as 79 per cent of some (Addis Ababa) urban populations live in conditions of extreme deprivation. As the twenty-first century begins, the urban poor represent a quarter of the total world population, caught up in a complex web of unemployment and chronic underemployment, poor pay, low education and malnutrition.[40] Some estimates have already placed the number of unemployed in developed countries at about 30 million, more than 70 per cent of them in urban areas. At least 220 million people in cities lack access to clean drinking water and it is estimated that 420 million have no access to the most simple of latrines.[41]

One of the more immediate results of this growing poverty in new urban centres is the range of new and old disease problems that are emerging in and around cities. In the 1970s, cities were still becoming safe havens against many diseases, but the combination of uncontrolled rural–urban movement and the ensuing poverty that has been created has made it possible for diseases that were previously close to being controlled to make a reappearance. The urbanization of rural parasitic diseases, for example, is a relatively new phenomenon that is being fostered by high population density, inadequate housing, poor sanitation and water supply. [42] Together with other social problems, they are rapidly undermining the capacity of people to break the cycle of poverty and under-development and are exposing people to more severe infections than might be the case for people living in endemic areas.

The poverty of conditions is affecting all health indicators however. In some low-income settlements in New Delhi, the child mortality rate is 221 per 1000 and nearly twice as high among the poorest of the poor. In urban areas of Guatemala, infant mortality rates vary from 113 per 1000 for children of illiterate women in the lowest socio-economic group to 33 per 1000 for children in more educated families.[43] In low-income areas in Karachi, between 95 and 152 infants per 1000 live births die before the age of 12 months. In the slums of Port-au-Prince, Haiti, where 1 in 5 infants die before the first birthday and 1 in 10 between the first and second birthdays, the urban rate is almost three times higher than in rural areas. The problem is clearly a multifaceted one that involves a mix of generalized lack of health care services, widespread poor health and nutrition, and low educational levels, in settings that are themselves becoming environmentally hostile.

Poor urban sanitation in and around overcrowded cities has made urban areas prone to mosquitoes and a variety of parasites. Problems of urban malaria, dengue and dengue hemorrhagic fever, and yellow fever[44] in cities such as Karachi,[45] Calcutta,[46] Madras,[47] Khartoum,[48] Dar es Salaam[49] and parts of Nigeria have become new public health challenges. Studies in Brazil[50] and Thailand and India[51] refer to the emerging role of massive rural–urban migration on the spread of visceral leish-maniasis, as well as the spread of malaria[52] and in Sudan the migration of people from drought-affected areas to Khartoum has been associated with a significant increase in cutaneous leishmaniasis.

How best to reach vulnerable groups in urban centres with the type and quality of health and social services needed, remains problematic. Investments in these sectors is going down rather than up, and even if there were more funds available, the pace of unplanned growth of urban populations in poor countries may well be exceeding the capacity of existing infrastructures to keep up with them.

Some of the experiences with the problem are nevertheless proving noteworthy. Cities such as Cali (Colombia), Jakarta (Indonesia), Karachi (Pakistan), Mexico City and São Paolo (Brazil) have initiated efforts to respond to the overcrowding and overload on central hospital facilities. By strengthening peripheral health units and training massive numbers of new staff who can be allocated to urban primary care facilities, some headway has been achieved.

Migration and health

Richer countries have been no exception to some of these changes, and have highlighted the complex economic and political nature of migration. Mass population movement within, between and into the European Union (EU) countries has become an increasingly vital part of the economic and political development of the bonds uniting them.

Migration is not new to countries of the EU, and throughout the first half of the twentieth century emigration continued to be an effective economic and social safety valve for most of them. As a net exporter of people, Europe benefited from mass emigration to the Americas, Australasia and, to a lesser extent, Africa. The second fifty years benefited equally from the ability of people to move internally and meet regional demands for a mobile labour force. The emergence of the EU as a new economic entity has nevertheless brought about radical changes in the nature and direction of migration, and it is now attracting migrants from developed as well as developing regions of the world. The emerging pattern is unlikely to change soon.

Tuberculosis is essentially a disease of poverty. It thrives where there is an absence of good nutrition, where housing is inadequate, and where overcrowding and poor ventilation are common.[53] Overall improvements in standards of living and in the quality of healthcare throughout much of Europe, and certainly in most EU countries, significantly reduced the incidence and prevalence of TB over the course of the past 50 years. The same economic progress has not been forthcoming in all parts of the world, and similar health benefits have failed to accrue in many poorer countries. In these, as well as in countries that have recently experienced wars and social upheaval, TB has remained a problem, and at a global level, there are signs that it could be on the increase again. In 1993, the World Health Organization (WHO) announced that TB had again become an emergency and predicted as many as 10 million new cases by the early part of the twenty-first century.

People arriving from poor countries are likely to be at higher risk of TB than non-migrants, and a number of EU countries are already seeing changes in their epidemiological profiles in the context of TB. In Denmark, the incidence of new cases has increased steadily over the past five years and the proportion of foreign-born cases rose from 18 per cent in 1986, to 60 per cent in 1996.[54] In England and Wales, approximately 40 per cent of all TB is estimated to occur in people from the Indian subcontinent[55] and in the Netherlands, where the incidence of TB rose 45 per cent between 1987 and 1995, over 50 per cent of known cases were among immigrants.[56] Similar TB profiles are being reported in Germany and France where migrants are three times and six times respectively more likely to be diagnosed with the disease than non-migrants.[57]

The problem, however, may not simply be one of the social conditions in which people lived prior to migration. The fact that they are often socially excluded and tend to remain economically disadvantaged are likely to make them prone to diseases of poverty.[58] This is particularly true for people arriving on short, temporary work permits, and those arriving 'unofficially', but it is by no means unique to these groups.

Labour migration often means concentrations of people in substandard housing where overcrowding and poor sanitation are common. This has been so in the Netherlands,[59] Austria[60] and France.[61] A study of migrant workers in the farming region of Almeria in southern Spain, found that 85 per cent of them were living in makeshift overcrowded accommodation juxtaposed to the greenhouses and warehouses they worked in. Over 75 per cent of the accommodation had no running water, 75 per cent had no toilet facilities, 70 per cent no electricity, 95 per cent no heating or air conditioning, and 65 per cent no refuse collection.

A study of living conditions among people from Cape Verde in Lisbon reported that most housing was illegal, and located on land that had not been allocated for construction or equipped with amenities. Over a third of the houses had no piped water; 19 per cent had no separate kitchen area, and 13 per cent had no bathroom or toilet facilities. In 26 per cent of the houses there was no organized sewage disposal and 13 per cent had no electricity.[62] A 1991 study of TB found that 13 per cent of the 622 new cases of TB were among migrants living in this area.[63] In Italy, where the pace of immigration has grown rapidly in recent years, substandard housing and poor access to public health services has also been highlighted by Italian health authorities as potential sites for the emergence of chronic and drug-resistant TB.[64] Interviews with Moroccan patients hospitalized for TB in France reflect the pervasiveness of poor housing among immigrants and its possible association with poor health including TB. [65]

Movement of people within and between countries has become a central theme of current day European Union society. It nurtures economic development, encourages interdependence between countries and regions, and also provides an important resource exchange link between the EU and other countries. There is a well-established economic need for this movement of human resources, and it is unlikely that the trend will diminish of its own accord in the foreseeable future. Indeed with time, the free movement of people that has now become a basic principle of the EU will no doubt be extended to include other countries as they are admitted to the Union.

Despite the magnitude of the challenge, relatively little attention has been given to the role of migration in changing the epidemiological profile of receiving communities, or on the impact migration and resettlement has on the health of migrants. Even less attention has been paid to the conditions that are possibly linked to the process of health development in the context of migration. National health statistics rarely reflect the process or its implications, and there has been relatively little interest in the phenomenon by health and social scientists. What data are available tend to be from small studies and anecdotal reports. They nevertheless suggest that the health circumstances that surround and characterize uprooting and migration merit more consideration.

Much of course depends on the type of population movement in question, why and where it occurs, and the profile of the people involved. However, the fact that most migrants move because of the 'push' of poverty rather than the 'pull' of alternative living conditions means that many of them inevitably come from socio-economically deprived backgrounds that are not able to provide a good quality of life or health. Migrants moving because of poverty come with predictable health profiles: poverty breeds the diseases of poverty, regardless of location or time in history.

The range of health outcomes that can be associated with migration is broad. It includes communicable and non-communicable physical diseases; injuries associated with the work environment; and psychological problems. All, or any, of them can be debilitating to the health of migrants and their families and have social and economic consequences for host countries as well as for migrants and their families.

The reality of migration within and into the EU today is one of changing and emerging trends in health. The association of health screening with the possibility of expulsion does little to encourage migrants to participate, and indeed may defeat the whole purpose of it. Unofficial migrants are possibly at particularly high risk of TB, and very reluctant to be tested for fear of legal measures. Screening for other diseases such as hepatitis B, which also constitutes a growing threat, could also be effective if it is done in a constructive way.

Culture conflict is also a common and serious problem in migration. It affects people in different ways, some more overtly than others. To what extent culture conflict or clash is linked to the mental health problems reported among migrants is not clear, but there is reason to believe that it is a factor. Just as with other health indicators, however, there is a paucity of information on the incidence and prevalence of mental health problems among migrants. What data are available suggest that cultural background plays an important role in predisposing some migrants to diseases such as depression, chronic anxiety, neuroses and schizophrenia. Alcohol abuse may also be a coping response gone wrong.

Conclusion

Population movements are now occurring on a scale rarely seen before. People are choosing or being forced to uproot and move in unprecedented numbers, and the geographic extent and speed of their movement is also growing rapidly. There are a number of reasons for this. A mass media system that cuts across countries and cultures has made it possible for people to know and think more about other societies and perceived opportunities. The emergence of a globalized economy and labour market has meanwhile required and encouraged a wider movement of work-related migration than at any other time in history. Better and easier transportation has made all of this easier to both conceive and implement.

There have also been major push factors. Population pressures and land scarcity in many parts of the world have come together to force people to search for a better living elsewhere. Wars and complex emergencies, especially but not only in poorer regions of the world, have displaced more people than ever before. Meanwhile there is mounting evidence that environmental development schemes, as well as environmental degradation, are also forcing people to move from their homes in unprecedented numbers.

In the past, migration has been thought of as a positive force in economic development, and indeed in some parts of the world this has been, and may still be, the case. People who move in search of work often succeed, are able to re-establish themselves and even support families back home. For many people, moreover, urban centres may still be seen as offering more opportunities than rural agricultural areas.

On the whole, however, the pace and magnitude of contemporary population movement is outpacing the capacity of many countries to cope. Uncontrolled urbanization is contributing to the emergence of vast shanty towns and slums that offer little relief from poverty, poor housing, insanitary living conditions, and overcrowding. The physical and social diseases associated with urban poverty are becoming a chronic problem that defies any easy or short-term solution.

At the same time, the number of people who have been, and no doubt will continue to be, displaced by political instability, complex emergencies and environmental change is also exceeding the capacity of many receiving countries and communities to meet the most basic needs of people. This is especially so when the countries in question are poor and already overburdened by weak social and health infrastructures. The capacity of, and justification for, humanitarian and development agencies to provide long-term support is also becoming a major concern.

Thus despite the potential that always exists for personal improvement through migration, serious public health, socioeconomic and political problems are emerging in many parts of the world as a result of population movement, and particularly so when these movements are poorly planned and/or managed. The epidemiology of urban disease is already changing as a result of rural–urban and circular migration, and the health of forcibly displaced people has become increasingly problematic as a result of the numbers of people concerned. The long-term social and economic impact may be even greater if migration to already overloaded cities begins to create an intergenerational cycle of poverty. Making population movement a healthy and constructive process is becoming a major challenge. The pace and size of the changes taking place has caught many countries and the international community as a whole poorly prepared, and it calls for policies and programmes that have not yet been developed. If sustainable development is to be fostered rather than undermined, new and visionary steps will have to be taken at all levels of national and international government. Population movement has become an integral part of modern society and development, but to date there has been little recognition of either this or the size of the phenomenon and its implications.

Notes

1 L. Diamond, *Promoting Democracy in the 1990s: Actors and Instruments, Issues and Instruments* (New York: Carnegie Commission on Preventing Deadly Conflict, 1995).
2 World Bank, *World Bank Lending for Large Dams: a Preliminary Review of Impacts* (Washington, DC: World Bank, 1996).
3 M. M. Cernea and S. Guggenheim, 'Performance: Influencing Policy and Reducing Displacement in Resettlement and Development', in *The Bankwide Review of Projects Involving Involuntary Resettlement 1986–1993* (Washington, DC: World Bank, 1996); UNHCR, *The State of the World's Refugees 1995: In Search of Solutions* (Oxford: Oxford University Press, 1995).
4 Food and Agriculture Organization (FAO), *The State of Food and Agriculture* (Rome: FAO, 1993); Food and Agriculture Organization (FAO)/World Health Organization (WHO), *International Conference on Nutrition and Development – a Global Assessment* (Rome: FAO/WHO, 1992).
5 A. Adepoju, *Emigration Dynamics in Sub-Saharan Africa: the Economic, Demographic, Political and Ecological Conditions and Policy Implications*. Discussion paper from a policy workshop held in Kampala on Emigration Dynamics in Sub-Saharan Africa, 4–5 December 1995 (Geneva: International Organization for Migration, 1995).
6 WHO, *Health Population and Development: WHO Position Paper: International Conference on Population and Development 1994, Cairo*. (Geneva: WHO, 1994); D. Satterthwaite, 'The Social and Environmental Problems Associated with Rapid Urbanization'. Paper presented at the Expert Group Meeting on Population Distribution and Migration, Santa Cruz, Bolivia, 18–22 January 1993; WHO, *Improving Urban Health: a Programme for Action* (Geneva: WHO, 1988).
7 J. S. Nabila, 'Population and Sustainable Development with Particular Reference to Linkages among Environment, Urbanization and Migration in ECA Member States'. Paper prepared for the United Nations Economic Commission for Africa, Series E/ECA/POP/TP/95/3(b) /3, 1995.
8 E. K. Mburugu, *A Resettlement Survey in the Kiambere Hydroelectric Power Project: Preliminary Report*, March 1988.

9   M. Toure and T. O. Fadayomi (eds), *Migrations Development & Urbanization Policies in Sub-Saharan Africa* (Oxford: Council for the Development of Social Science Research in Africa, 1992).

10   B. G. Swapna, 'Involuntary Migration and the Associated Schism: Case of a River Valley Project in India', *Journal für Entwicklungspolitik*, 11(3) (1995) pp. 349–63; S. Jain, 'Habitat, Human Displacement and Development Cost: a Case Study', *Social Action*, 45(3) (1995) pp. 299–317; T. Scudder, 'Development-Induced Relocation and Refugee Studies: 37 Years of Change and Continuity among Zambia's Gwenbe Tonga', *Journal of Refugee Studies*, 6(2) (1993) pp. 123–52; S. C. Varma, *Human Resettlement in the Lower Narmada Basin* (Bhopal: Government Central Press, 1985).

11   T. O. Fadayome, S. O. Titilola, B. Oni et al., 'Migrations and Development Policies in Nigeria', in M. Toure and T. O. Fadayome (eds), op. cit.; S. Maimouna, A. Ba and N. Ndiaye, 'Demographic Implications of Development Policies in the Sahel: the Case of Senegal', ibid.; B. Zaba and J. Clarke (eds), *Environment and Population Change* (Liège: IUSSP, 1992).

12   World Bank (1996), op. cit.

13   M. M. Cernea and S. Guggenheim, op. cit.; G. Parent, A. Ouédraogo, N. M. Zagré et al., 'Large Dams, Health and Nutrition in Africa: Beyond the Controversy', *Sante*, 7(6) (1997) pp. 417–22; J. P. Nozais and M. Gentilini, 'Les Conséquences sanitaires du developpement economique des pays tropicaux', *Tropical Medicine*, 45(1) (1985) pp. 73–8.

14   A. Jouan, B. Le Guenno, J. P. Digoutte, et al., 'An RVF Epidemic in Southern Mauritania', *Annals of the Pasteur Institute of Virology*, 139 (1988) pp. 307–8; J. Walsh, 'Rift Valley Fever Rears its Head', *Science*, 240 (1988) pp. 1397–9.

15   G. Parent, A. Ouédraogo and N. M. Zagré et al., op. cit.

16   M. J. Toole and R. J. Waldman, 'Prevention of Excess Mortality in Refugee and Displaced Populations in Developing Countries', *Journal of the American Medical Association*, 263(24) (1990) pp. 3296–302.

17   International Centre for Migration and Health (ICMH), *Migrants, Displaced People and Drug Abuse: a Public Health Challenge* (Antwerp: ICMH, 1998).

18   J. Macrae, A. Zwi and V. Forsythe, 'AIDS Policy in Transition: a Preliminary Analysis of the "Post"-Conflict Rehabilitation of the Health Sector', *Journal of International Development*, 7(4) (1995) pp. 669–84.

19   Handicap International, *The Problematic of Landmines*. Abstract from www.creativem.com/handicap/Conf 01.htm. (1997).

20   Personal communication, Rui Gama Vaz, June 1998.

21   J. Macrae, A. Zwi and L. Gilson, 'A Triple Burden for Health Sector Reform: "Post"-Conflict Rehabilitation in Uganda', *Social Science and Medicine*, 42(7) (1996) pp. 1095–108.

22   M. J. Toole and R. J. Waldman, op. cit.

23   M. J. Toole and R. J. Waldman, 'An Analysis of Mortality Trends Among Refugee Populations in Somalia, Sudan, and Thailand', *Bulletin of the World Health Organization*, 66 (1988) pp. 237–47.

24   ICMH, op. cit.; M. Carballo, S. Simic and D. Zeric, 'Health in Countries Torn by Conflicts: Lessons from Sarajevo', *The Lancet*, 348 (1996) pp. 872–4.

25 M. Carballo, M. Grocutt and A. Hadzihasanovic, 'Women and Migration: a Public Health Issue', World Health Statistics Quarterly, 49 (1996) pp. 158–64; Carballo et al., ibid.; ICMH, op. cit.

26 Goma Epidemiology Group, 'Public Health Impact of Rwandan Refugee Crisis: What Happened in Goma, Zaire, in July, 1994?' The Lancet, 345 (1995) pp. 339–43.

27 A. Naficy, M. R. Rao, C. Paquet et al., 'Treatment and Vaccination Strategies to Control Cholera in Sub-Saharan Refugee Settings: a Cost-Effectiveness Analysis', Journal of the American Medical Association, 279(7) (1988) pp. 521–5.

28 Centers for Disease Control and Prevention (CDC), 'Famine-affected, Refugee, and Displaced Populations: Recommendations for Public Health Issues', Morbidity and Mortality Weekly Reports, 41 (1992).

29 M. J. Toole and R. J. Waldman, op. cit.

30 P. Shears, A. M. Berry, R. Murphy et al., 'Epidemiological Assessment of the Health and Nutrition of Ethiopian Refugees in Emergency Camps in Sudan', British Medical Journal, 295 (1987) pp. 314–18.

31 M. J. Toole and R. J. Waldman, op. cit.; Shears and Lusty, op. cit.; C. Aall, 'Disastrous International Relief Failure: a Report on Burmese Refugees in Bangladesh from May to December 1978', Disasters, 3 (1979) pp. 429–34.

32 M. J. Toole and R. J. Waldman, ibid.; United Nations Childrens Fund (UNICEF), State of the World's Children (Oxford: Oxford University Press, 1985).

33 M. Carballo, S. Simic and D. Zeric, op. cit.

34 M. J. Toole and R. J. Waldman (1990), op. cit.; C. Hasselblad, C. Davis and R. Waldman, First Report of the CDC Epidemiologic Team to the Somali Ministry of Health (Atlanta: Centers for Disease Control, 1980); P. Shears, A. M. Berry, R. Murphy et al., 'Epidemiological Assessment of the Health and Nutrition of Ethiopian Refugees in Emergency Camps in Sudan', British Medical Journal, 295 (1987) pp. 314–18.

35 ICMH, op. cit.

36 World Health Organization, Health and Urbanization in Developing Countries: Discussion Note. Expert Group Meeting on Population Distribution and Migration, Santa Cruz, Bolivia, 18–22 January 1993. (ESD/P/ICPD.1994/ VG.VI/INF.8, 1994).

37 Ibid.

38 Ibid.

39 Ibid.

40 T. Harpham and C. Stephens, 'Urbanization and Health in Developing Countries', World Health Statistics Quarterly, 44(2) (1991) pp. 62–9.

41 World Resources Institute (WRI), World Resources 1996–1997 (Washington, DC: WRI, 1996).

42 Harpham and Stephens, op. cit.

43 Ibid.

44 N. Gratz and J. Hamon, 'Ecology and Vector Control', Interdisciplinary Science Review 3(3) (1978) pp. 214–19.

45 D. R. Nalin, F. Mahmood, H. Rathor et al., 'A Point Survey of Peri-Urban and Urban Malaria in Karachi', Journal of Tropical Medicine and Hygiene 88 (1985) pp. 7–15.

46   S. P. Mukhopadhyay, 'Resurgence of Malaria with Special Reference to Malaria Outbreak in Calcutta', *Journal of the Indian Medical Association* 94(4) (1996) pp. 145–6.

47   B. Hyma, A. Ramesh and K. P. Chakrapani, 'Urban Malaria Control Situation and Environmental Issues, Madras City, India', *Ecology of Disease* 2(4) (1983) pp. 321–35.

48   Rayah et al., 'Competition between *Culex quinquefasciatus* Say and *Anopheles arabiensis* Patton in the Khartoum Area, Sudan', *International Journal of Biometerology*, (1983).

49   C. F. Cortis and R. G. Feachem, 'Sanitation and *Culex pipiens* Mosquitoes: a Brief Overview', *Journal of Tropical Medicine and Hygiene*, 84 (1981) pp. 17–25.

50   S. M. B. Jeronimo, R. M. Oliveria, S. Mackay et al., 'An Urban Outbreak of Visceral Leishmaniasis in Natal, Brazil', *Transactions of the Royal Society of Tropical Medicine and Hygiene*, 88 (1994) pp. 386–8.

51   N. K. Sethi, Y. Choudri and C. S. Chuttani, 'Role of Migratory Population in Keeping Up Endemicity of Malaria in Metropolitan Cities in India', *Journal of Communicable Disease*, 2 (1990) pp. 86–91.

52   A. Cruz Marques, 'Human Migration and the Spread of Malaria in Brazil', *Parasitology Today*, 3(6) (1987) pp. 166–70.

53   M. D. Almeida and J. E. Thomas, (1996). 'Nutritional Consequences of Migration', *Scandinavian Journal of Nutrition*, (40)2 (Suppl. 31, 1996) pp. 119–21; H. L. Rieder, J. P. Zellweger, M. C. Raviglione et al., 'Tuberculosis Control in Europe and International Migration', *European Respiratory Journal*, 7 (1994) pp. 1545–53.

54   F. Prinsze, 'Tuberculosis in Countries of the European Union', *Infectieziekten bulletin*, 8(2) (1997) pp. 25–7.

55   G. Karmi, 'Migration and Health in the United Kingdom', in A. Huismann, C. Weilandt and A. Geiger (eds), *Country Reports on Migration and Health in Europe* (Bonn: Wissenschaftliches Institut der Ärzte Deutschlands e.V., 1997); 'National Survey of Tuberculosis Notifications in England and Wales in 1983: Characteristics of the Disease', *Tubercule*, 68 (1987) pp. 19–32.

56   J. de Jong and R. Wesenbenk, 'Migration and Health in the Netherlands', in Huismann, Weilandt and Geiger, ibid.

57   M. Gliber,(1997) 'Migration and Health in France', in ibid.

58   WHO (1996), ibid.; O. S. Gaspar, 'Migration and Health in Spain', in ibid.

59   J. de Jong and R. Wesenbenk, op. cit.

60   G. Hammer, '*Lebensbedingungen ausländischer Staatsbürger in Österreich*', in *Statitische Nachrichten* (11/94) pp. 914–26.

61   M. Gliber, op. cit.

62   Almeida and Thomas, op. cit.

63   M. J. Gardete and M. Antunes, 'Tuberculose em Imigrantes: estudo preliminar em sete serviços de tuberculose e doenças respiratorias dos Distritos de Lisboa e Setubal', *Saude em Numeros*, 8(4) (1993).

64   F. Carchedi and A. Picciolini, 'Migration and Health in Italy', in A. Huismann, C. Weilandt and A. Geiger (eds), op. cit.

65   S. Nejmi, 'Social and Health Care of Moroccan Workers in Europe', in M. Colledge, H. A. van Guens and P. G. Svensson (eds), *Migration and Health: Towards an Understanding of the Health Care Needs of Ethnic Minorities* (Geneva: WHO Regional Office for Europe, 1983) pp. 138–49.

3

Case Studies of Infectious Disease Outbreaks in Cities: Emerging Factors and Policy Issues

Debarati Guha-Sapir

Introduction

The increasing concern for deteriorating health situations in the major urban areas of the developing world today is belated. Signs of burgeoning urban populations caused by increasing rural–urban migration and natural increase among the already urbanized community were evident in the past decade and earlier. Recent regressing conditions in rural areas have caused individuals and families to move to cities faster than ever in the hope of a solution to their plight. This hope keeps the urban migrants in the degrading conditions that the city offers them and continues to attract others. There are many estimates of growth in cities around the world. Throughout the world, rapid increases in urban populations of up to 66 per cent and have been projected and as much as 100 per cent in tropical and sub-tropical countries. The main contribution to this increase comes from megalopolises in Latin America and South Asia. For example, New Delhi, Bombay and Calcutta in India fall within the sixteen fastest growing cities in the world. Their growth rates are 125, 88 and 75 per cent respectively to the end of 1999.

An important factor in the consideration of health status of urban populations is their essential heterogeneity. This heterogeneity is at the base of two characteristics that have influenced health policies and strategies in urban centres and will continue to do so for some time to come. First, the concentration of people who are economically better off in cities has necessarily biased the distribution of health facilities and quality of care in their favour. The visibility and political influence of the upper-class city inhabitants have systematically drawn health resources to the city in nearly all developing countries in the world today. Urban health systems therefore have been largely modelled on advanced western systems built to serve the upper socio-economic classes, whose epidemiological profile resembles that of the western communities. As a result, the focus for international and national health and development agencies has justifiably shifted to rural communities as areas where the need for support was critical. The primary health care approach was conceived with rural traditional communities as a target. Despite this attention, concentration of wealth in cities has engendered the concentration of health resources in urban areas.

The second factor influencing the general appreciation of the health situation in cities has been significantly better indices of health and nutritional conditions in urban than in rural populations. It has been persuasively demonstrated, with increasing evidence, that these indices are misleading. Aggregated city health statistics usually look much better than rural ones. These better rates reflect the economically privileged section of the metropolis whose epidemiological profile is frequently not very different from that of the average western population. Averaging the extreme differences in health status between the squatter and the upper-middle-class person successfully camouflages the gravity of the problem among the urban poor. The numerator of such indices is biased in favour of the well-off, since most of the urban poor are not part of any official health system and the denominator is, on the other hand, expanded by their presence. The issue of urban health draws its criticality today largely with regard to the urban poor. Housing and habitation can influence prevalence and susceptibility to specific infectious diseases. Numbers of slum and shanty dwellers, squatters, pavement dwellers and the homeless are growing in almost every Third World city. In certain cities, they represent the predominant class of inhabitants. Their increasingly visible presence is finally attracting the attention of local and national authorities, if only as a source of risk to the rest of the city inhabitants.

Background

Before beginning a discussion on epidemics in cities, it is useful to clarify the context in which some of the epidemics discussed have occurred. Most major metropolises of the developing world have witnessed an exponential increase in their urban poor. Slum dwellers and squatters account for 60 per cent in Kinshasa (Zaire), 46 per cent in Mexico City (Mexico), 67 per cent in Calcutta (India), 55 per cent in Manila (Philippines) and

79 per cent in Addis Ababa (Ethiopia). Calcutta leads the group with over five million people living in slum or substantially worse conditions. In most other cities the numbers of urban poor are over one million. The larger portion of this growth is due to natural increase of the population, which Harpham[1] estimates at 61 per cent of the total increase. The other 39 per cent she attributes to migration.

The conditions of life of these urban poor groups are the predisposing factors for disease outbreaks and epidemics in almost laboratory conditions. Environmental conditions resemble those in eighteenth and nineteenth century Europe. Open sewers, uncollected rubbish, poor sanitation, flies, standing water and poor lighting, along with the 'benefits' of industrialization and modernization, such as pollution, toxic wastes, bottled drinks and processed foods have created conditions where increased susceptibility and rapid transmission of disease are greatly increased.

Other aspects of urban life can further aggravate the disease pattern of an individual or group. Crowding and promiscuity afford excellent opportunities for the transmission of infection. The city family has, curiously enough, remained as large as in rural traditional situations. Studies in Calcutta, Bombay and Hyderabad slums reveal a mean family size (persons eating out of the same kitchen) of over six members. While family size has carried over, traditional support structures have failed. Conditions in urban slums do not provide opportunities for kitchen gardens or the cultivation of small plots of land.

The two-parent family and the presence of elders essential to child care and supervision has disintegrated. Working hours and patterns have radically changed from the rural system. As a result, households are more frequently headed by a single mother working as a domestic servant or as a day labourer at a construction site. The hours of work in domestic service cover the better part of the day and evening, during which the children remain without supervision of care. Defecation and washing habits are neither inculcated nor guided, greatly increasing the risk of gastro-intestinal infections and all other faecally transmitted diseases. The use of convenience foods such as soft drinks and packaged or fried snacks further lower the nutritional status of the child and set the stage for the proliferation of disease. Prevalence of breast-feeding is often low due to difficulties in taking the infant to work (normal in the fields in rural areas) and baby foods are substituted. The implications of food substitution and early weaning of the child for diarrhoeal diseases have been extensively and persuasively discussed in the literature. In a study aimed at identifying social and environmental factors associated with the risk of child mortality in a peri-urban community in The Gambia, children of employed women were found to be at increased risk of dying. The women worked in the informal sector, selling and trading fruit, vegetables or cooked food. Although the children did not appear to be more economically disadvantaged compared with the other co-habitants, the risk could be attributed to lack of maternal care.

Mortality in the early stages of life in a Porto Allegre study has consistently shown significantly higher rates of infant neonatal and post neonatal mortality among slum children compared to non-slum dwellers.

Systematic lack of appropriate health services for those working in the informal sector and those disenfranchised or homeless can aggravate outbreaks. Differentials in the epidemiological profiles and susceptibilities among migrants into the city compared to the inhabitants are also risk factors for increased disease occurrence and transmission.

Urban patterns of infectious diseases: an overview from mortality data

Our understanding of the pattern of infectious disease in cities suffers from a remarkable dearth of studies to evaluate the effects of urbanization or urban risk factors in the transmission and susceptibility of disease. An important piece of work on urban mortality was undertaken by the Inter-American Investigation of Mortality in 1967 and 1973[2] in which data were collected from 15 project areas for childhood mortality and 12 cities for total mortality. While some cities from industrialized countries were included, 10 of the twelve cities were in Latin America. Unfortunately, the dynamics of urbanization in Latin America have made the data collected for this report largely outdated by now. In addition, all the weaknesses attendant on the use of mortality data in developing countries contribute to reducing the utility of the study. However, it is of great value as it is the only one of its kind in the health sector undertaken in a systematic manner and at a time when the issue was not recognized as a priority by the health authorities.

The study reported on 12 cities: Bogota, Bristol, Cali, Caracas, Guatemala City, La Plata, Lima, Mexico City, Ribeira Preto, San Francisco, Santiago and São Paulo. The pattern of infectious diseases based on the mortality statistics of selected cities reveals a wide variation among them. In general, cities with high mortality from a particular disease tended to have high mortality from all other infectious and parasitic diseases. The infectious disease groups included in the study follow, with those diseases subject to epidemics mentioned in parentheses: tuberculosis, intestinal infections (typhoid fever; other salmonella infections; bacillary dysentery; amebiasis; food poisoning); other infective and parasitic diseases (tetanus, infectious encephelitis, infectious hepatitis, malaria); respiratory diseases (influenza). Death rates from tuberculosis were substantially higher in males than females in almost every age group with the highest rates being noted in Lima and Santiago. In the latter city, the death rate from this disease was nearly twice as high as the next highest (Peru) and three times as high as the third ranking cities. The increase in death rates in Santiago was manifested among persons 35–54 years of age, whereas in most other cities the death rates increase after the age of 54 years. Variation in the rates among the cities is considerable and wide disparity is noted. It is evident that the epidemiological behaviour of fatal tuberculosis in these cities differed markedly and in a complex manner. This is not surprising in view of the many factors that affect incidence as well as mortality of a disease such as tuberculosis. Communities differ in pressures of infection, in risks of exposure, the levels of immunization, the adequacy of control measures and the efficacy of therapy. Migration of individuals susceptible to the disease into the city could explain some of the high mortality. In São Paulo, 22 of the 55 deaths occurred among relative newcomers to the city; however, this was not consistently observed in every city. Quality of death registration and reporting systems as well as diagnosis of the cause of death varies from city to city. This makes cross-city comparisons extremely hazardous. Intestinal infections, which are considered the scourge of urban slums and particularly susceptible to outbreaks, account for relatively lower death rates compared to the other diseases. Guatemala City displayed the highest death rates from all intestinal infectious diseases. When examined more closely, Mexico City registered the highest level of deaths due to amebiasis with Guatemala ranking second. It is customary to regard intestinal infections as reliable indices of the sanitary state of the environment. Earlier, disease-specific mortality might have been as useful as disease incidence. With the modern methods of specific therapy, it would be advisable to obtain reliable morbidity data before drawing inferences about sanitary conditions in these cities.

Among other infective and parasitic diseases, infectious hepatitis caused the largest number of deaths. Bogota and Lima accounted for nearly half the deaths. Although no hard data were readily available for this study, China has also expressed preoccupation with frequent outbreaks of infectious hepatitis in many cities, due principally to food contamination and poisoning.

Death rates from respiratory diseases were markedly higher among males than females. The ratios of male to female deaths was about 2 to 1 in all of the cities except Bogotá and Cali. Santiago presented the highest death rates for influenza and pneumonia in both males and females. The excessive mortality of men in age group 35–54 in Santiago and Mexico City (67.4 and 43.8 per 100 000 respectively) may have been related to a high prevalence of cirrhosis of the liver due to alcoholism. Clinicians have long maintained that the prognosis of pneumonia in the alcoholic subject is poor and that he is more likely to contract that disease.

Diarrhoeal diseases deserve a special place in a discussion of urban environmental factors and infectious disease outbreaks. Diarrhoea is the most frequent primary and secondary cause of death in developing countries, yet is the most responsive to the environmental and sanitary conditions which characterize urban living conditions of the poor.

The fallacies of rural urban statistics have been convincingly demonstrated by many authors in recent years. Basta[3] has pointed out that intra-urban differences may be greater than those between rural and urban areas and are not reflected in urban averages. Data from the above mentioned Inter-American Investigation on Mortality present comparative statistics on death rates from diarrhoeal diseases (per 100 000) among children 0–5 years old. With the exception of Brazil (Recife) and Jamaica (Kingston), mortality figures are consistently higher in the rural population than the urban. This type of comparison may well represent a selection effect or the misleading result of aggregating data over the entire urban population, thus diluting the denominator.

The lower death rates from intestinal infections may be explained by the variability of reporting and under-registration. Moreover, these diseases are frequently not the immediate cause of death. If underlying causes are not recorded, diagnosis of these diseases may never occur.

One study showed that the prevalence of campylobacter excretion in children aged 6–59 months in one poor urban and one rural community was 44.9 and 28.4 per cent respectively. The prevalences were inversely related to the quality of water supply. The difference was maintained in children who had diarrhoea at the time of the sample collection (45 and 33 per cent) or a history of diarrhoea (41 and 26 per cent). Campylobacter was the bacterial organism most prevalent in these children and was positively correlated with the presence of helminths (85.6 and 66 per cent in urban and rural communities). Ninety-four per cent of urban children over 2.5 years of age harboured helminths. It was postulated that poor hygienic conditions and heavy soil contamination in the urban slums were responsible for chronic helminthic infestation. This then creates a niche for campylobacter. In another similar study by

Cole[4] in The Gambia, diarrhoeal disease prevalence in the urban site of the study was estimated at 18.7 per cent compared to 11.8 per cent in a comparable rural site. A survey of the prevalence of *Escherichia coli* as an aetiological agent of infantile diarrhoea in Ghana[5] showed similar infection rates in urban populations in Accra (6.5 per cent) and in a rural community. In this study, however, specimens were taken from children attending an urban polyclinic and a rural health centre and may not provide an accurate picture of the prevalence in the population at large.

These studies serve to underline the potential importance of infectious disease, particularly diarrhoea, in urban slum conditions. The lack of data from the slum populations and their marginalization from social, legislative and welfare systems severely bias the existing information. In the very recent past, however, emergency situations resulting from epidemic outbreaks of meningoccocal meningitis in sub-Saharan Africa and severe floods in Bangladesh and Brazil have provided the opportunity to examine specific dimensions of epidemic disease in urban environments.

Cholera epidemics in urban agglomerations: the case of Dhaka, Bangladesh

Bangladesh is a tropical country comprising the delta of three major rivers which drain a total area of 16 million square kilometres. Forty per cent of the country is one metre below sea level and over half the country is at risk of floods. Bangladesh lies in a geographic area prone to cyclones, floods and droughts. The country has a population of 106 million with a crude growth rate of the urban population at 7.6 per cent per annum. Infant mortality is 139 per 1000 and child mortality is 205 per 1000 in children under five.

Floods occur at regular intervals in the deltaic plains of Bangladesh, usually followed by significant increases in diarrhoeal diseases including cholera. Until 1963, the classic *Vibrio cholerae* biotype was observed in both India and Bangladesh, but in 1966, *El tor* biotype first appeared in Bangladesh. By 1973, all cholera cases were due to the *El tor* biotype and in 1974 and 1975 the biggest cholera epidemic ever recorded in Dhaka occurred. The epidemiology of the *El tor* biotype differs from that of the classic *Vibrio cholerae*. The peak incidence of *El tor* cholera has been reported to occur one month earlier than the classic *Vibrio* in Bangladesh, although the epidemic in 1974 was close to the traditional peak periods of October and November following the monsoons and in this year the floods.

Following the 1971 war of independence in Bangladesh (previously East Pakistan), thousands of homeless and unemployed flocked to Dhaka for government assistance. A severe food crisis in 1973 and heavy floods in 1974 seriously affected the country. The homeless and the jobless built huts and shelters near the markets, railway tracks, industrial parks, city outskirts and unused public lots. These settlements had no waste disposal facilities; few and distant handpumps were available. Residents typically used water from rivulets, ponds and canals for bathing, washing and drinking. This set the stage in Dhaka for future epidemics.

Modes of cholera transmission have been abundantly researched and urban epidemics in Bahrain, Italy, Malaysia, the Philippines and Portugal have been studied.[6] Specific urban factors related to the transmission of the disease have been relatively few. Transmission factors seem to apply to both rural and urban conditions.

There have been several important cholera epidemics in urban Bangladesh. One of the earliest studied by the Cholera Research Laboratory (now International Centre for Diarrhoeal Disease Research) was the epidemic of 1962–3. The only study of this epidemic reported index cases and rates of transmission to family contacts. The transmission rates among families of male index cases were observed to be lower (12 per cent) than when the index case was female (39 per cent). About 70 per cent of family contacts became ill within three days of the index case.[7]

Martin et al.[8] analysed a classic cholera outbreak in 1964. The epidemic peaked several times over many months and was usually localized. The analysis was almost exclusively restricted to an examination of index cases and their transmission patterns. Very little attention was given to factors determining the localization in time and space. Again, female index cases had higher rates of transmission to family contacts than male index cases.

The epidemic of 1974 occurred in October and had the dubious distinction of being the largest ever recorded. In Dhaka hospitals, 993 cases of cholera in children aged 60 months and younger were recorded. An interesting issue regarding urbanization effects in this study is that it compares the effects of types of eating places of the cholera victims on control individuals in a matched pair analysis. Persons who ate at charitable feeding centres and roadside food stalls were at significantly higher risk of contracting the disease than those who ate at home. The famine of 1973 and the earlier war brought a large influx of migrants to Dhaka. Free meals were distributed by voluntary and government agencies. The price of food in the city had skyrocketed. Thousands of people depended on the feeding centres. Contamination of the cooked food and drink by unhygienic preparation and handling of the food could easily have set off a major epidemic.

Other results of the urban concerns of the study contradicted former evidence of high-risk age groups. The literature traditionally identifies young male adults as being at greatest risk. In this Dhaka study, the high-risk age group was clearly children under nine years of age (49 per cent of all cases). These high rates should be interpreted with care since it is unclear whether the results were due to low vibrocidal titres in children or if children were hospitalized more often than women or adults in general.

Adult females are at special risk. They generally avoid going to hospitals, but are more frequently exposed since they nurse and clean the sick, launder soiled clothes and wash faeces from children.

Studies of cholera outbreaks in other urban centres have provided disparate insights into urban living and risks of outbreak. General sanitary conditions and water scarcity are principal risk factors of outbreaks. An excess of water (flooding for example) will not normally produce an outbreak since there will be a greater dilution of the pathogen. In addition, during the outbreak in Portugal (in Lisbon and other parts of the country), commercially bottled mineral water was implicated in the epidemic. A series of epidemiological studies on cholera transmission in the slums of Calcutta was carried out in the mid-1960s.[9] The study sampled water sources and latrines to test for the presence of *Vibrio cholerae*. During the ten-month sampling period, 46 per cent of the latrines were positive for *V. cholerae*. Nearly all the isolates from the latrines were *V. cholerae* or *El Tor*. The study population normally used bucket type latrines (93 per cent). Subsequently, a detailed investigation of an outbreak was undertaken by the Joint Indian Council of Medical Research-Government of West Bengal-World Health Organization Cholera Study Group[10] in a slum of Northern Calcutta. Fourteen shanty families were surrounded by better-class housing. Each family lived in one room and used a portion of the common corridor for cooking, washing and eating. Water was collected from a public tap and a tube located far outside the community. Garbage and faeces were deposited in the central corridor. The main mode of transmission of infection was clearly the extreme unsanitary conditions of housing and living patterns.

The 1970 cholera outbreak in Jerusalem was characterized in the early phases by widely scattered sporadic cases, often in males. It began in the third week of August and peaked 29 August to 26 September. The important role of family contacts evinced in the studies in Dhaka and

Calcutta was not observed here. The contamination was traced to individuals returning to suburban Jerusalem, from the neighbouring countries where active cases were known. The night soil used for vegetable cultivation was subsequently contaminated by these returnees. Jerusalem was the principal market for the contaminated vegetables. Once there were infections and cholera cases in Jerusalem, the city sewage became contaminated and this contaminated vegetables irrigated by sewage in the outskirts of the city. These contaminated vegetables were sold in city markets, maintaining the cycle of transmission. No solid evidence was presented for this hypothesis but it was considered plausible.[11]

A study of the cholera outbreak in Bahrain in August–October 1978 reported an increased relative risk of cholera in bottle-fed infants over infants who were breastfed (9 times). No difference was found for other factors, such as solid food intake, water storage, frequency of bathing, use of soap, maternal cholera infection or water source. A low economic status and inadequate diet were noted as the principal characteristics of the cholera patients admitted to hospital in Manila during the 1961 outbreak.[12] Twenty-six of the 27 autopsied cases had ascariasis, with very heavy loads of worms. High prevalence and intensity of ascariasis are indicative of poverty, and result in faecally contaminated yards and lanes. Similarly, in the 1973 outbreak in Colombo, Sri Lanka, most of the cases were poor people living on the banks of the Kelani river. The river was found to be bacteriologically contaminated. On the basis of this physical association with a cholera-prone community and a polluted river, it was concluded that the river population served as a focus of cholera dissemination in Colombo.

In conclusion, outbreaks of cholera in cities have been associated with unhygienic and unsanitary conditions related to faecal habits and waste disposal. Densely packed living quarters and crowding have resulted in deposits of excreta in and around eating and washing areas. Contamination of water sources used for drinking and washing and also for irrigation can set off infection. Mass food distributions or commercial feeding centres and stalls can be responsible for epidemic diseases. Roadside food stalls and bottled water have been the source of contamination. Migration into cities and settlements in poor neighbourhoods can carry infection and infect a whole community. Finally, women, in their tasks of caring for the sick, laundering and cleaning soiled clothes and sick children are at higher risk of contracting cholera. Breastfeeding infants reduces the risk of infection in babies, whereas bottle feeding increases it. Yet in the urban context, the type of occupation and working hours of poor women tend to discourage breastfeeding.

Meningitis epidemic of 1988 and 1989 in sub-Saharan Africa: the cases of Addis Ababa, Khartoum and N'Djamena

In Africa, meningococcal meningitis constitutes a serious health problem causing high mortality and morbidity. Of all causes of cerebrospinal meningitis, meningococcal meningitis is the most disturbing for the international community. The infection is characterized by epidemics which create emergency situations not only in the country where the epidemic occurs, but in the neighbouring countries and beyond. The semi-arid region south of the Sahara and south of the equator has been called the 'meningitis belt'. In this area, endemo-sporadic infections occur annually in the dry season, while large-scale epidemics occur at longer intervals. An Expert Consultation in 1983 emphasized the importance of effective surveillance, which was to serve two purposes: the detection of the epidemics' onset and activation of response; and the evaluation of control measures.

Since then, two related problems have been identified. One, prediction of an outbreak, has been deficient, since the epidemic is not recognized until it is well under way. Two, early warning indicators (not strictly related to a surveillance system but to environmental factors such as rainfall, wind patterns and migration) have been hypothesized but remain untested. Patterns in the behaviour of the epidemic which are obvious in smaller unit analysis pose questions in the definition of the risk factor of an epidemic. A large geographic area might disguise or misrepresent the nature of the spread and obfuscate the risk factors related to it. A study on the epidemic of meningococcal meningitis in Ethiopia, Sudan and Chad in 1988 and 1989 focused on the capital cities simply as densely populated urban conglomerations particularly vulnerable to the rapid transmission of meningococcal meningitis and as areas where the bulk of the cases occurred. The latter consideration is coloured by the possibility that case-reporting in the rural areas is less efficient and the higher case load in cities could be a statistical artefact. However, it is generally admitted that the observed distribution of the cases in these epidemics is consistent with the known risk factors for epidemic forms. The data for the study were collected although the analysis is not yet complete. The following therefore is a summary of the overview of the situation as presented by the data.

The study collected three types of data for the metropolitan areas of Addis Ababa, Khartoum and N'Djamena: information based on interviews with the health authorities and other responsible officers involved in the epidemic; recorded data from hospitals serving the metropolitan area in past epidemics; and data on reported cerebro-spinal meningitis (CSM) cases on non-epidemic years. The entire data collection covered a period of four weeks in September 1990.[13]

Sudan: Khartoum

Sudan lies in the eastern section of the 'meningitis belt' and is the country with the first recorded epidemic, at the end of the nineteenth century. In 1950–1, the country experienced a devastating epidemic with more than 50 000 cases reported. The 1988 and 1989 epidemics reported 38 805 cases (2770 deaths) with most cases falling in the 1988 peak. Meningitis is a notifiable disease in the Sudan and there is a Central Epidemiology Unit for specific disease surveillance.

In January 1988 the first cases of the epidemic were registered in the outskirts of Khartoum. The disease rapidly spread through the three sections of the city – Khartoum, Khartoum North and Omdurman. More than a third of the total number of cases occurred in Khartoum city. By mid-February, the emergency system was alerted and thereafter data were collected daily. Although underestimation of cases reported to the emergency system was significant (indicated by a special study of three major hospitals during the month of February), the trends of the epidemic were sufficiently reflected by the data in the epidemiological system. The number of cases increased threefold per week until the peak was reached in the sixth week of the epidemic, when 1519 cases were recorded in Khartoum. In March, 52 samples were analysed in the Central Laboratory of Khartoum showing *N. meningitis* Group A. All samples were sensitive to sulfadiazine, crystalline penicillin, ampicillin and chloramphenicol, although a survey in May 1988 revealed resistance to sulfadiazine. In March, schools, cinemas and stadiums were shut down and messages were broadcast through the media.

Mass vaccination (using polyvalent A and C meningococcal polysaccharide vaccine) was begun in the third week of February and the 60 existing Expanded Programme of Immunization (EPI) centres of the capital city were brought into action. Approximately sixty to eighty thousand persons were vaccinated each day. Due to famines and civil strifes, Khartoum has recently seen a substantial increase in its urban poor. These are mainly destitute families from the countryside who have migrated to the capital for food and employment. In areas where the displaced populations were settled, the vaccination coverage was much lower than in the general population. This was due to a lack of EPI centres, health infrastructure and lack of mobility of the mobile teams.

Although the detection of the epidemic was rapid, response was comparatively slow. A lack of preparedness included an absence of instruments and no means of data collection and compilation. In addition, inadequate assessment of the epidemic's magnitude and the needs for control resulted in a full-blown epidemic.

Ethiopia: Addis Ababa

The western part of Addis Ababa lies in the Lepeyssonnie meningitis belt. It has experienced several epidemics, including a severe one in 1981 with 38 700 reported cases. Traditionally, Gondar, Gojjam, Wollo, Wollega, Shoa and Eritrea are the areas at high risk of CSM outbreaks. Meningitis is a notifiable disease in Ethiopia, with a weekly collection system. The first cases of the last epidemic were reported from Addis Ababa in November 1987. In December, 17 cases were reported and an alarm was sent to a city hospital (Ethio-Swedish Paediatric Hospital). Specific measures in Addis Ababa were initiated at the end of January 1988 and the increase in the number of cases peaked in February. Active case detection began in the *kebeles* (small administrative units within the city) where cases had been reported and only Rifampicin chemoprophylaxis was provided to household close contacts. In February, the strategy became more aggressive, with immunization for all high risk groups (all persons less than 20 years of age in schools, prisons and military camps, including health workers) and by April nearly 70 000 persons were vaccinated.

Chad: N'Djamena

Chad falls well within the 'meningitis belt' and experienced two epidemics of CSM in the 1980s. The 1988 epidemic began in February in N'Djamena, but unlike the other two countries, no outbreak occurred in 1989. Meningitis is a notifiable disease in Chad as in the other countries and is reported monthly. Cases of CSM among children under five years of age (16.4 per cent of the population) are not reported and therefore the number of cases entering the surveillance system can be significantly biased. The 1988 epidemic in N'Djamena began with the first cases in February. The Central Hospital is the major hospital of the city and received almost all the patients of the city, the patients arriving at its emergency ward. Since the hospital was the exclusive treatment centre of the cases, delay in the declaration of the epidemic in the city was very short. During this first month the numbers in the hospital increased dramatically and by 22 February an epidemic was declared. Most of the cases were from the city itself and some from the surrounding northern areas.

The Comité d'Action Sanitaire d'Urgence (CASU) took measures to contain the epidemic in the city and made an effort to diffuse congestion in the Central Hospital by opening three other peripheral centres. Resources, however, were concentrated or were only available at the Central Hospital. Peripheral centres provided only ambulatory treatment and were open only during normal daytime working hours. No doctor attended these centres. As a result, cases tended to come to the Central Hospital. A vaccination campaign was begun in early February for high-risk groups, largely dictated by the costs of accessing the group for vaccination purposes. In 11 days, 119 500 high-risk persons and 37 000 non-targeted persons were vaccinated in the city. This preferential vaccination caused some violence, aimed at the vaccinators and at the general policy. The high-risk targeting was not well directed and there was a recurrence of the epidemic after a temporary reduction in the number of cases.

Leptospirosis outbreak following floods in São Paulo

Leptospirosis outbreaks have been noted in the cities of São Paulo and Rio de Janeiro since the beginning of this century. The more recent epidemics occurred in São Paulo in 1983 (383 recorded cases) and 1987 (340). In Rio de Janeiro, a massive outbreak of more than 700 cases was recorded after the heavy floods in 1988. The link between flooding and epidemics of leptospirosis has been noted by several authors. The risk of an outbreak increases substantially by the concurrence of several factors: floods, population density, presence of rats, cats and dogs and the incidence of animal leptospirosis.

The study summarized here was undertaken in São Paulo following the floods of late 1987. It interviewed 107 patients and examined their domestic environment. These leptospirosis cases were diagnosed with serological confirmation at the University of São Paulo Hospital and infection was traced to their homes.[14]

The Municipality of São Paulo has witnessed uncontrolled urban sprawl in the last few years and the *favela* or shanty towns stretch endlessly on the outskirts of the city. Fifteen million people live within the city limits and the population continues to grow exponentially. Due to this growth, large areas of fertile land have been covered over by concrete effectively making these areas impermeable to water and promoting uncontrolled channelling of rainwater. The sloping terrain and natural embankments towards the River Tiete which passes by the north of the city have been filled and raised to increase building land.

This has aggravated the deficient drainage of water. The atmospheric pollution and geophysical conditions linked to the vast number of persons living in the city have altered the microclimate and meteorological pattern in the region. The Tiete River has been entirely canalized and a dam was constructed that artificially raised the level of the river. Following heavy rainfall, the city experiences frequent microflooding – that is, small collections of water in low-lying areas of the city. An increase in the incidence of leptospirosis has been noted regularly following city flooding. The results of the study clearly showed that environmental risk factors are related to the occurrence of the disease. Ninety per cent of the leptospirosis cases were male which reinforces findings from other studies. This sex distribution has generally been explained by the increased risk of occupational exposure to contaminated waters.

In this study, nearly half (48.8 per cent) of the cases reported contact with flood waters in their homes prior to the onset of the symptoms. Of all the cases, 48.7 per cent lived on the edges of the main roads leading out of the city and the rest in slums, colonies or by the edges of unpaved roads. Nearly 70 per cent of the cases lived less than 200 metres from an unused or abandoned lot and 38.5 per cent lived less than 200 metres from a city or council garbage dump. The presence of rats and stray dogs was noted in both the lots and the garbage dumps.

All of the cases consulted a physician upon the development of symptoms and nearly all were hospitalized. Approximately 10 per cent developed renal insufficiencies and were treated with dialysis. The average length of hospitalization was 10.6 days.

The direct costs of hospitalization of more than 1000 man-days (not including related costs of medicines and services in addition to the expensive intervention of dialysis) add up to a substantial amount. The repeated occurrence of these floods and the consequent increase of leptospirosis in the city should militate for measures to prevent outbreaks or merely control it at an early stage. Measures to eliminate rats and stray dogs should be used as strategies for long-term effects and would be cheaper than providing curative services to all the leptospirosis cases. Furthermore, an alert service to sensitize the public health physicians working within the (clearly) functioning health care system would encourage earlier diagnosis and reduce complications from the disease. The cost-effectiveness of veterinarian, sanitary and epidemiological measures should be estimated for a rational strategy to control the outbreaks of the disease.

Other factors mediating risk of disease outbreaks in urban settlements

Despite limited literature on the spread of infectious diseases in urban areas, certain factors clearly stand out as important in the development of strategies for the future.

Inequalities in distribution of health resources within cities

Studies are necessary to examine the phenomenon of the masking of severe health problems of the urban poor by the healthy urban majority. These studies must control for differentials related to income, housing quality and standard of living. There have been few such studies dedicated to contrasting the health and epidemiological profiles of the urban rich versus the urban poor. Such studies would pinpoint the nature of risks and the epidemiological profile of the vulnerable groups, rather than drawing assumptions from studies which do not adequately control for these factors.

One pertinent study undertaken in Mexico City examined differential health status within the city boundaries between the upper economic classes and the urban poor.[15] The author noted that the prevalent diseases in the slums of Mexico were largely infectious respiratory diseases, namely bronchitis, tuberculosis, influenza and pneumonia. He also noted the regular occurrence of intestinal disorders such as enteritis and other diarrhoeal diseases. Typhoid and paratyphoid were also common. The high incidence of intestinal infections amongst localized groups within city limits has been observed in several studies. It has been demonstrated that those living in 'irregular' settlements in the eastern suburbs of Netzahualcoyotl were especially sensitive to poor water supply and sanitary conditions.

A high prevalence of infectious disease among the urban poor has been documented in many studies. In his Mexico study, Ward examined a factor that mediated the use of health services by the sick inhabitants of the lower-class urban areas. He concluded that distance to a centre was a primary deterrent to the use of health services. A trade-off exists between losing a work-day and salary to get to a health facility, waiting in line, getting the prescription filled and letting the illness take its course. Medical treatment was the loser. He also found that if they did seek treatment, the sick would use a neighbourhood private practitioner with reasonable fees. It has also been noted that the extent to which low-income groups are obliged to make use of private sector health care when a public service exists is proof of inadequate service provided by the government sector. Spatial analyses of health centres in cities are clearly indicated in urban planning projects.

Acute respiratory infections and indoor air pollution

Between four and five million children under the age of five die in the world each year from acute respiratory infections (ARI). Most of these children are in developing countries. ARI studies have focused on the important issues of microbial causative agents, case management of antibiotics and effectiveness of vaccination. Research on risk factors has been judged to be less important, in spite of the dominance of risk-factor reduction in the history of ARI control in developed countries.[16] In developing countries, domestic air pollution has been assumed to be an important risk factor for ARI but there are very few studies examining this relationship.

ARI constitutes a serious threat to child survival in India. More than ten out of 1000 pre-school age children die of ARI in India. The situation is particularly discouraging among urban children. Community level studies have shown a magnitude of 5–7 episodes per year among urban children and 3–5 episodes among rural ones. Although the ARI group of diseases have varied aetiology, a large number of the risk factors are preventable at community and individual levels. The implications of ARI in children include chronic obstructive airway diseases as they reach adulthood. The National Institute of Communicable Diseases (NICD), India, estimated that among malnourished children, the relative risks due to pneumonia and bronchitis are 19 and three respectively. In addition to the high infection rate among malnourished children, lack of cellular immunity increases the disease rate, the incidence of secondary illnesses and the duration of illness. All these factors aggravate malnutrition. The NICD also reports on passive smoking as a risk factor for ARI. They found that the incidence of pneumonia and bronchitis in the first year of life was associated with parents' smoking habits. In addition they point out the high risk in urban housing where indoor pollution caused by wood, charcoal and coal fires contributes to an increase in the incidence of these diseases.

These particularly elevated levels of acute respiratory illnesses in urban slum populations have also been noted in Calcutta. This increase in respiratory infections was noted following the slum improvement project which provided flats to the shanty dwellers. The two-room apartments in high-rise blocks were conceived for a family to live and sleep in one room and cook in the other. These were rapidly transformed to flats housing two families, one in each room. Thus cooking on open coal fires occurred in the two rooms: the room designed to serve as the kitchen with ventilation and drainage, and the living room without these facilities. The health centre staff in the slum operated by the All India Institute of Public Health rapidly observed a rise in respiratory infections and identified the cause. But no suitable solution was formulated at that time. The alarming levels of indoor air pollution in the slums of Calcutta are apparent to the casual observer. There are street-level habitations with heating and cooking in unvented space. The ambient pollution of industrial waste, coupled with road traffic and various forms of disgorgement into the atmosphere does not require refined studies to establish that there is serious pollution.

The common fuel used by most slum inhabitants in Calcutta is biomass which contains significant amounts of the most serious pollutants – carbon monoxide, particulates, hydrocarbons and, to a lesser extent, nitrogen oxides. Smoke from coal (the other popular fuel) contains all of the above in addition to sulphur oxides, organic ash particles, and heavy metals such as lead. A study in Ahmedabad,[17] found a statistically significant higher incidence of respiratory infections and lung abnormalities in women. The investigators suggest that the prolonged exposure of women to cooking fuels is the cause of this higher level of disease. In China, coal combustion has been the prime source of urban atmospheric pollution. In Shanghai, about half the population use coal-cake stoves for cooking.

The influence of indoor air pollution on immunological function was investigated in primary school children exposed to coal smoke at home and at school. Results were reported by Wang and Chen,[18] where children from coal-burning households showed a mean reduction of white cell count of 13 per cent and 50 per cent transfer of lymphocytes.

The evidence presented by Chen and researchers in India argues strongly that indoor air pollution is a risk factor for acute respiratory infections. The total population exposed to high concentrations of smoke and other pollutants amounts to several hundred million. Very few epidemiological studies on pollution have been undertaken considering its seriousness today and greater concern for the future. The importance of ARI as an important cause of early childhood mortality and morbidity in many developing countries and serious prevailing indoor pollution make this issue one of high priority.

Conclusions

Irrespective of the country or the continent, health experiences are similar in most major cities of the developing world. The lessons learnt could apply to many of them and allow for improvement of health.

There are a few clear conclusions to be drawn from the above discussion, although it should be emphasized that not many epidemiological studies have been undertaken for the express purpose of identifying urban risk factors in the outbreak of infectious disease. Thus, the first conclusion to be drawn is that the problem must be adequately defined and understood before strategies can be proposed. The factors interlinking urbanization with attendant environmental concerns and psychosocial health problems provide diverse influences on the health conditions of a population. Although there is little reliable information, health trends seem to point in a few clearly discernible directions. From the perspective of infectious disease control and the responsibility of the health sector, the following five issues should be considered in future policy development:

The influx of new people

Migrants, refugees, victims of natural disasters or job hunters who come into a city increase environmental pressure and heighten the risk of disease outbreaks in different ways. The host population may be susceptible to an imported disease; and the arriving population may be extremely susceptible to an endemic disease which can very easily set off an epidemic of serious dimensions.

Food contamination

Contamination, especially at food stalls or distribution centres, can be an important source of infection and disease outbreaks. Due to the nature of urban living, common eating places and commercially produced food are more a part of everyday life than in rural areas. Changes in food habits due to working patterns among women heighten not only the vulnerability of bottle-fed infants but also that of young children on a diet of bottled drinks and snacks.

Women

Urbanization imposes upon underprivileged women multiple responsibilities of livelihood and family care. This places them at higher risk of contracting the diseases discussed above. In turn, they could then generate increased transmission of the disease in the community. In addition, their role influences several critical aspects in a child's life which can affect its vulnerability to infectious diseases.

Lack of sufficient parental care

This absence of adequate care, especially in single-parent homes (increasingly common among the urban poor), engenders unhygienic defecating and washing habits and adds to the risk of disease transmission and pollution.

Health surveillance and monitoring systems

The surveillance and monitoring systems in these cities precisely exclude the population groups who are most susceptible to outbreaks and who form the focal points in most epidemics. The lack of expertise in epidemiological principles in health offices retards recognition of an epidemic and reduces the capacity to propose effective control measures. In most cases where the surveillance systems are functional, they operate based on select institutions whose patient populations are not those amongst whom outbreaks occur. It is only when the outbreak reaches the marginal populations and grows to proportions which affect the entire population that health systems recognize it and react. In addition, at the action level, the presence of logistical infrastructure and the legitimacy of housing will determine the distribution of control measures. Frequently the peak of the epidemic is missed. Epidemic control actions are often oriented towards the wrong location; they miss the places where the index cases begin. Sometimes the health actions miss the areas where the majority of cases are located. Vaccinations in schools, the military, prisons and organized institutions effectively exclude those subgroups of the population most susceptible to the disease. These subgroups then become responsible for transmission and continuation of the epidemic. Mapping of the cases, for example, in a metropolitan area, would quickly identify geographic areas at risk. In situations of limited resources, mass vaccination coverage of at-risk areas could possibly be an effective mechanism to control the spread of the disease.

The evidence in the literature, though limited, points to an urban health profile distinctly different from that of a classic rural community. The core health problems among the urban poor are faecally transmitted diseases, airborne diseases and malnutrition. These three elements interact cumulatively and synergistically to produce volatile conditions in terms of disease transmission. The situation in slums can be effectively compared to refugee camps. Camps have a high incidence of tuberculosis and different forms of conjunctivitis. There are frequent outbreaks of measles, meningitis and malaria if the displaced persons travel from highlands or non-endemic areas to malarious regions. Similar to reports from refugee camps, epidemics of vector borne diseases such as dengue fever and filariasis have been recorded in urban slums associated with the accumulation of water in iron drums and rubber tyres.[19]

All the usual environmental risks which undermine health status apply to outbreaks of diseases. Housing density and sexual promiscuity increase the risk of disease transmission in the usual ways. Environmental sanitation including control of flies, mosquitoes and rats will further reduce the risk. Stray dogs and cats, rarely mentioned, should occupy a priority place in environmental cleaning programmes to eliminate vectors. Any visitor to Calcutta and Bombay cannot deny the potential played by these animals as they scavenge in the garbage heaps and the slum living quarters. They can transmit and encourage disease and vermin. Water supply and excreta disposal remain critical priorities. These have the greatest potential in controlling disease.

But a fundamental measure that should be considered for the success of any epidemic or infectious disease control is social legislation. Social legislation is the key to recognition by city authorities of those populations most susceptible to disease and thus the initial focal epidemic cases. The tautological situation in many cities occurs because infectious diseases and risk of epidemics remain highest among the very groups which, due to their 'illegitimate' existence (refugees, migrants, homeless) do not have the right to health and sanitary services. This typically gives rise to a self-defeating situation in which the control of diseases in the larger city population becomes nearly impossible since a human ecological niche is ignored. As the burden of these populations grows in the cities, the problem of infectious diseases and control of outbreaks will become increasingly acute.

The advent of AIDS has had the 'salutary' effect of forcibly emphasizing the need to provide health services to everyone in the community, if the entire community is to survive. The experiences in the meningitis study, the initial phase of the Calcutta slum study, and the Mexico City study on distribution of health facilities underscore the importance of equitable health services in all cities. The chances that policies will change in this direction are reasonably strong since the effects of the voids are felt by populations who have, so far, been protected from the depressing poverty of rural areas.

Finally, health strategies for control of infectious diseases and epidemics in cities should first recognize that the problem is rooted among the urban poor. Any plan should be oriented towards this group. Efforts to enact social legislation to legitimize their existence is fundamental to the success of a health action plan. An 'ostrich' approach to migrants, displaced persons or pavement dwellers will only increase the risk of disease. Within a narrower framework, it is clear that sanitary measures, in particular excreta disposal and lavatory facilities, could be the most effective input. Non-structural approaches towards the same objectives should also be considered including education of mothers and school children about hygienic excretion. Surveillance systems that monitor high-risk groups can be the key to early recognition and control of impending outbreaks. In this context, epidemiological training for health and sanitary officers, including the veterinary service, would enhance the performance of such a system. Geographic methods, such as the mapping and spatial analysis for spread of disease and the planning of health services, would contribute significantly towards the funnelling of health resources to the crux of the problem. Indirectly, health services for working women, especially single mothers and their children, would improve conditions that predispose these communities to outbreaks.

Notes

1 T. Harpham, 'Health and the Urban Poor', *Health Policy and Planning*, 1 (1) (1986) pp. 5–18.
2 R. R. Puffer and C. V. Serrano, *Patterns of Mortality in Childhood, Report of the Inter-American Investigation of Mortality in Childhood* (PAHO, Scientific Publication No. 262, 1973).
3 S. S. Basta, 'Nutrition and Health in Low-Income Urban Areas of the Third World', *Ecology and Food Nutrition*, 6 (1977) pp. 113–24.
4 T. J. Cole, 'Relating Growth Rate to Environmental Factors: Methodological Problems in the Study of Growth-Infection Interaction', *Acta Paediatrika Scandinavika Suppl.*, 350 (1989) pp. 14–20.
5 D. Abgodaze, C. A. Abrahams and S. Arai, 'Enteropathogenic and Enterooxigenic *Escherichia Coli* as Aetiological Factors of Infantile Diarrhoea in Rural and Urban Ghana', *Transcriptions of the Royal Society of Medicine and Hygiene*, 82 (1988) pp. 488–91.
6 Khan et al., 'The El Tor Cholera Epidemic in Dhaka in 1974 and 1975', *Bulletin of the World Health Organization*, 61 (4) (1983) pp. 653–9.
7 R. Oseason et al., 'Clinical and Bacteriological Findings among Families of Cholera Patients', *Lancet* (1996) pp. 340–2.
8 R. Martin et al., 'Epidemiologic Analysis of Endemic Cholera in Urban East Pakistan', *American Journal of Epidemiology*, 89 (1969) pp. 572–82.
9 R. Sinha et al., 'Cholera Carrier Studies in Calcutta', *Bulletin of the World Health Organization*, 37 (1967) pp. 87–100.
10 Joint ICMR-GWB-WHO Cholera Study Group, 'Study on *V. Cholerae* Infection in a Small Community in Calcutta', *Bulletin of the World Health Organization*, 43 (1970) pp. 401–6.
11 R. G. Feacham, 'Environmental Aspects of Cholera Epidemiology: a Review of Selected Reports of Epidemic and Endemic Situations during 1961–1980', *Tropical Disease Bulletin*, 78 (8) (1981) pp. 675–98.
12 C. K. Wallace et al., 'The 1961 Cholera Epidemic in Manila, Philippines', *Bulletin of the World Health Organization*, 30 (1964) pp. 795–810.
13 D. Guha-Sapir and F. Hariga, 'An Epidemiologic Analysis of Cerebro-Spinal Meningitis Outbreaks in Urban Agglomerations: the Cases of Addis Ababa, N'Djamena and Khartoum' (in manuscript).

14 D. Guha-Sapir and A. Lombardi, 'Retrospective Study of Leptospirosis Cases Registered in the Municipality of São Paulo between 20/12/87 and 20/3/88' (1989).

15 P. Ward, 'Reproduction of Social Inequality: Access to Health Services in Mexico City', *Health Policy and Planning*, 2 (1) pp. 44–57.

16 H. Chen et al., 'Indoor Air Pollution in Developing Countries', *World Health Statistics Quarterly*, 43 (1990) pp. 12–138.

17 Reported by Chen et al., op. cit.

18 Ibid.

19 A. Benyyoussef, J. L. Cutler, R. Baylet et al., 'Santé Migration et Urbanisation', *Bulletin of the World Health Organization*, 49 (1973) pp. 517–37.

4

The Role of International Law in the Control of Emerging Infectious Diseases

David P. Fidler

Introduction

Physicians, scientists, and public health officials the world over recognize the emergence and re-emergence of infectious diseases as one of the great public health challenges for humankind at the approach of the new millennium. Emerging infectious diseases (EIDs) pose problems of enormous scale and complexity for those who practice the healing art. Those who have been leading the counterattack against EIDs also recognize that these diseases raise serious issues for those who practice the political and legal arts. To address EIDs effectively will require translating what is scientifically and medically necessary to combat pathogenic microbes into feasible political and legal action. This translation process will be particularly evident and difficult in connection with international law. Translating epidemiology into international law will require an active interdisciplinary discourse between infectious disease experts and international lawyers. Such a discourse is only now in its formative stages, and this chapter attempts to stimulate its development by providing an analysis of the role of international law in the control of EIDs.

My analysis begins with a brief explanation of why international law is critical to plans to deal with the EID threat. The chapter then provides a historical overview of the role of international law in the control of infectious diseases. I next evaluate the existing international law on infectious disease control. I then briefly discuss other areas of international law that touch on infectious disease control. The review next examines current developments in international law stimulated by the

EID problem. Finally, I offer some educated guesses about the future directions international law may take as the EID saga continues to unfold.

The need for international law

International law can be briefly defined as the rules regulating the behavior of states in the international system. The sovereign states in the international system make and apply the rules of international law. The primary sources of international law are treaties, customary international law, and general principles of law recognized by civilized nations[*1] because these sources emanate directly from the actual conduct of states.[2] Subsidiary sources of international law include national and international judicial decisions and the writings of the most highly qualified publicists of the various nations.[3] These are subsidiary sources because they interpret rules made directly by states through, for example, a treaty or custom.

This brief description of international law provides the first reason why international law is critical to attempts to deal with the global EID problem: the world is structured into independent sovereign states that recognize no common, higher authority. In such an anarchical system, only the states themselves can regulate their conduct; and international law is the historical product of state interaction in a decentralized, anarchic environment. The driving force for international law is state consent. The critical need for international law is not, therefore, peculiar to the EID problem because no issue escapes the basic structure of the international system.

The second reason why international law is critical to EID plans flows from the nature of the EID threat. The problem of the emergence and re-emergence of infectious diseases is considered by experts to be a global problem: one that no single state can deal with independently.[4] More specifically, EIDs undermine a state's sovereignty by making it virtually impossible for a state to provide for its public's health without the cooperation of other nations.[5] EIDs contribute to the globalization of public health, which can be defined as the denationalization of public health policy, in the sense that states are losing control over their national public health conditions in the face of global forces.[6] In this regard, the EID problem is related to such phenomena as the globalization of markets. National and international public health officials have recognized the reality of the globalization of public health in their arguments that the traditional distinction between national and international public health is no longer valid.[7] To provide for public health in the era of EIDs, states are forced to cooperate through diplomacy and international law.[8]

Efforts to combat EIDs must utilize international law for structural and substantive reasons. This conclusion is not novel from a historical perspective, as the critical role of international law in infectious disease control has been recognized since at least the mid-nineteenth century, when states first sensed the globalization of public health.[9] Grasping the importance of international law to infectious disease control today may not be difficult. What is often harder for people to understand or accept is the limited potential of international law to improve international relations.[10] One of the most frequent criticisms about international law is its ineffectiveness because states sometimes choose not to comply with or enforce its rules. This ineffectiveness stems largely from the structure of the international system. International law is both indispensable and sometimes ineffective. This combination of characteristics forces us to approach the role of international law in infectious disease control with healthy caution.

The historical development of international law on infectious disease control

As mentioned earlier, international law has been important to international infectious disease control strategies since the mid-nineteenth century. In this section, I briefly present the historical development of the international law specifically concerning the control of infectious diseases. Understanding this development will provide historical perspective to the international legal challenge presented by EIDs.

Prior to the mid-nineteenth century, states combated the spread of infectious diseases unilaterally through the strategy of quarantine.[11] When the first international sanitary conference was held in 1851, states had begun to realize the ineffectiveness of quarantine policies as well as their adverse impact on growing international trade. The start of infectious disease diplomacy in 1851 marked states' understanding of the need for international cooperation on infectious disease control. The dominance of quarantine as a disease control strategy meant that customary international law on infectious disease control did not place affirmative duties on states to cooperate or restrict the kinds of measures states could take to keep diseases out of their territories. Treaties became, therefore, the international legal mechanism through which international cooperation on infectious diseases would be translated into international law. Various states conducted ten international sanitary conferences (1851, 1859, 1866, 1874, 1881, 1885, 1892, 1893, 1894 and 1897) and concluded four treaties on infectious disease control prior to the end of the century (1892, 1893, 1894 and 1897).[12] The 1903 International Sanitary Convention represented the first major breakthrough for the emerging international law on infectious disease control because it superseded the earlier treaties, set forth detailed provisions on dealing with the international spread of plague and cholera, and set in motion the process that led to the creation of the first international organization devoted to health.[13] Treaty-making on infectious disease control accelerated in the first half of the twentieth century as states adopted 13 more agreements that either amended the 1903 Convention, focused on regional efforts or addressed specific transportation technologies.

A detailed analysis of these treaties is beyond the scope of this chapter. The fundamental elements of the international legal regime on infectious disease control can, however, be found in the major treaties of this period. This international legal regime had three pillars: (1) duties to notify other states of outbreaks of specified diseases; (2) limits on the measures other states could take against the ships and aircraft coming from states experiencing disease outbreaks; and (3) involvement of an international organization dedicated to health.

One of the first responsibilities of the newly created World Health Organization (WHO) after the Second World War was to unify the separate international sanitation treaties in a single code. WHO adopted the International Sanitary Regulations in 1951, which replaced the previous set of treaties among member states of WHO. The International Sanitary Regulations were amended a number of times in the 1950s and 1960s and renamed the International Health Regulations (IHR) in 1969.[14] The IHR were last substantively revised in 1973 and were amended in 1981 to remove smallpox from the list of diseases subject to the Regulations.[15] Today, the IHR represents the 'only international health agreement on communicable diseases that is binding on Member States [of WHO]'.[16]

Evaluating existing international law on infectious diseases

EIDs have stimulated new analysis of the effectiveness of the IHR. In this section, I briefly present a critique of the existing international law on infectious diseases by analysing the substantive law from within each possible source of international law (Table 4.1).

Table 4.1   Sources of international law and their historical importance in the control of infectious diseases

Source	Historical importance
International agreements	Very important because international agreements have been the main source of international law on infectious diseases
Customary international law	Although a great deal of state practice exists to analyze for rules of custom, the analysis has never been done. Rudimentary analysis suggests no duty to notify disease outbreaks to other states and no limitations on measures taken against disease outbreaks in other states
General principles of law recognized by civilized nations	Not very important because principles of public health law generally applicable within states do not translate well into rules for relations between states
Judicial decisions	Not very important because there are no international judicial decisions that consider international legal rules on infectious disease control
Writings of the most highly qualified publicists of the various nations	Not very important because very few international lawyers have paid any attention to international law on infectious disease control
Soft law	The International Health Regulations could be interpreted as soft law because states do not treat them as binding obligations, and WHO prefers to operate through non-binding recommendations

International agreements on infectious disease control

International lawyers generally consider international agreements and customary international law to be the two most important sources of international law.[17] As illustrated earlier, international agreements are the most important historical source of international law on infectious disease. In this regard, international infectious disease control law has developed similarly to international economic law and international environmental law, both of which are heavily treaty-based.[18] International agreements are binding only on those states that become party to them.[19] The prominent place occupied by the IHR suggests that international agreements will continue to play a critical function in infectious disease control.

The IHR's objective is to ensure maximum protection against the international spread of disease with minimum interference with world traffic.[20] The IHR adopt the basic framework developed by the earlier sanitary conventions: (1) specific disease outbreak notification requirements; (2) limitations on the reaction of other states to notified disease outbreaks; and (3) leadership provided by an international health organization.[21] On none of these items can the IHR be considered successful. WHO officials and international legal scholars agree that member states of WHO have failed to make the IHR an effective international legal regime.[22] Throughout the history of the International Sanitary Regulations and the IHR, WHO member states have often failed to notify WHO of outbreaks of diseases subject to the Regulations.[23] As a result, the surveillance system intended to operate through the IHR has not worked properly, undermining the goal of maximum security against the international spread of disease. In addition, WHO member states have often taken restrictive trade and travel measures against other member states experiencing disease outbreaks that exceed the measures permitted by the Regulations.[24] Consequently, this behavior undercuts the goal of minimum interference with world traffic. Finally, despite notable successes like the eradication of smallpox, WHO has not made the progress against infectious disease that original proponents of the international health organization expected.[25] Although it remains central to international health activities, WHO suffers from financial constraints and political limitations created by its member states.[26]

The EID problem has accentuated all the weaknesses of the Regulations mentioned above, as well as exposing the inadequate scope of the Regulations' coverage of only three diseases (plague, cholera and yellow fever).[27] The recognized inadequacy of the Regulations has forced member states of WHO to begin the process of revising them to improve the international legal regime on infectious disease control,[28] which revision is discussed below (pp. 76–9). States are writing yet another chapter in the development of international agreements on infectious disease control.

Customary international law

A rule of customary international law exists when state practice is general and consistent in the international system and such practice is accompanied by a sense that it is required by international law.[29] Evidence of state practice can be found in many different places: diplomatic correspondence, policy statements, treaty practice and votes in multilateral fora.[30] A rule of customary international law binds all states, except those that persistently object to the rule's formation.[31] Rules of customary international law tend to be more general than rules that appear in treaties.[32] Examples of rules of customary international law include the immunity of diplomatic agents and freedom of navigation on the high seas.[33] Although customary international law is a more controversial source of international law than international agreements, it remains central to the modern system of international law.[34] Even though international agreements have dominated international law on infectious disease control, the long history of state practice on this issue should yield much material for customary international law analysis. It does not appear, however, that such an analysis has ever been undertaken.

Given the emphasis on the duty to notify disease outbreaks that appear consistently in the major international agreements from the 1903 International Sanitary Convention to the IHR, one might analyze this duty to notify, to determine whether it is a rule of customary international law. Not only might state practice support such a claim but it would also be bolstered by the general international legal principle of state responsibility that requires that states notify other states about possible dangers or harms emanating from their territory.[35] This line of reasoning does not, however, stand up after detailed analysis.

First, the frequent failure of states to fulfill the duty to notify, as witnessed under the IHR, erodes the argument that states generally and consistently notify other states about disease outbreaks. It also hurts the idea that states believe that such notifications are required by customary international law. Second, the claim that the duty to notify is customary international law does not focus on a critical question: what infectious disease does the duty cover? If the customary law duty to notify disease outbreaks tracks the limited scope of the notification duty in the IHR, then the customary duty suffers the same inadequate coverage as the existing IHR. Given that the IHR and its predecessors have determined the scope of the duty to notify disease outbreaks, state practice evidencing a broader notification duty covering more diseases with the potential to spread internationally is not likely to exist. Third, any purported customary law duty to notify does not address to whom exactly the duty is owed. Does a state experiencing a disease outbreak have to notify just neighboring states, more distant states with which it engages in extensive trade and travel, or the entire international community?

These questions all raise the issue whether customary international law is capable of generating rules on infectious disease control.

Another issue that complicates customary international legal analysis is the reciprocity of duties central to the international agreements on infectious disease control. States that receive disease outbreak notifications have the reciprocal duty not to take excessive measures against the trade and travel from the notifying state. In other words, the duty to notify and the duty not to deploy excessive measures are a 'package deal' because one cannot be separated from the other: a state is less likely to notify others of disease outbreaks if it is not assured that the other states will not act in ways that damage its economy in response to the notification. The argument that there is a duty to notify under customary international law without the reciprocal duty not to apply excessive measures can only be justified under the general principle of state responsibility rather than under customary law on infectious disease control because state practice for the latter is conditioned by the package deal. Whether or not state behavior under the IHR, for example, demonstrates a general and consistent practice supported by a sense of legal obligation not to apply excessive measures would have to be analyzed; but the historical record offers much state practice that would not support the existence of a customary rule prohibiting reactive measures that go beyond what is permitted by the IHR.

In summary, the content of customary international law on infectious disease control today is probably the same as it was in the mid-nineteenth century: there is neither a duty to notify other states of disease outbreaks beyond the vague duty imposed by the principle of state responsibility nor a duty to limit the actions taken in response to disease outbreaks in other states.

General principles of law

The third primary source of international law is 'general principles of law recognized by civilized nations'.[36] The legal principle that no one can be a judge in his own case has been referred to as a rule of international law or a 'general principle of law'.[37] This is not a widely used source of international law,[38] and it seems ill-suited to generate international law in the infectious disease context. Although most countries have laws that relate to public health, it is not clear that a survey of all jurisdictions would yield general principles of public health law applicable to international relations. Perhaps such a survey would reveal the importance of notifications of disease outbreaks by local physicians or authorities to central public health agencies. General principles of law might in that case support the notification duties that exist in international agreements or under customary international law, but it does little to create a distinct rule of international law on infectious disease control. In addition, looking to general principles of law would also have to take into account differences among the various states on what diseases are reportable. Once analysis starts to take into account such specific details of domestic legislation, it has moved away from *general* principles of law.

Judicial decisions

An important subsidiary means of determining rules of international law is to analyze national and international judicial and arbitral decisions that discuss international law.[39] Judicial and arbitral forums assist states in settling disputes. Given the breakdown in compliance with the IHR, one might expect member states of WHO to have much need of dispute settlement mechanisms. Judicial and arbitral decisions from international tribunals and domestic courts addressing IHR disputes are, however, non-existent. Nor are there any cases in which tribunals attempt to apply customary international law on infectious disease control.

The barrenness of case law on the international rules on infectious disease control suggests a couple of hypotheses. First, the lack of such case law might indicate that informal dispute settlement procedures, like good offices and mediation, successfully resolve disputes. The IHR dispute settlement procedure involves three consecutive steps for resolving a dispute: (1) referral of the dispute to the WHO Director-General; (2) if the WHO Director-General cannot resolve the dispute, then it can be referred to an appropriate committee of WHO; and (3) if referral to an appropriate committee fails to resolve the dispute, then any of the member states concerned may refer the dispute to the International Court of Justice.[40] While the WHO Director-General and the Committee on International Surveillance of Communicable Diseases have each resolved disputes, no IHR dispute has ever reached the International Court of Justice.[41] The scale of non-compliance with the IHR compared against the few disputes referred to the WHO Director-General suggests a second possibility: WHO member states do not seek to enforce their rights under the IHR. They neither activate the dispute settlement provisions of the IHR often nor enact countermeasures against states that violate IHR duties. Measures taken in excess of those permitted in the IHR might be seen to be countermeasures against a state that failed to notify a disease outbreak, but is not clear that state practice responding to failures to notify under the IHR actually acknowledges this legal reasoning. In addition, to be a lawful countermeasure, excessive measures taken in response to a failure to notify as required by the IHR would also have to satisfy the requirements for countermeasures under international law: notice, proportionality, and temporariness.[42] Again, states, in their practice, do not seem to employ countermeasures reasoning to justify their reactions to disease outbreaks in other states. Moreover, the countermeasures argument does nothing to justify excessive measures taken after a state notifies WHO in compliance with its IHR duty.

Writings of publicists

Another subsidiary means of determining rules of international law is to analyze the writings of the most highly qualified publicists of the various nations.[43] Practicing and academic international lawyers often produce valuable analysis of rules of international law that help states and tribunals understand them better. Unlike many areas of international law, the control of infectious diseases has not historically attracted the attention of many international lawyers. More international legal writings on infectious disease control are appearing with the advent of the EID threat.[44] Perhaps as awareness of the international legal challenges of EIDs grows the writings of publicists will become a more important resource than it has been historically in the area of infectious disease control.

Soft Law

In many ways, the existing international law on infectious disease control resembles what has been called in other international legal contexts 'soft law'.[45] Soft law occupies a zone that exists between morality and binding law. Soft law has been used to describe aspirational documents like resolutions of the United Nations General Assembly as well as provisions in treaties that demand little from states or that states do not obey. Although the IHR are technically binding rules, most states view them as merely recommendations rather than real obligations.[46] This attitude also helps explain why WHO member states do not routinely enforce their rights under the IHR. It also ties into the prevailing ethos at WHO that emphasizes non-binding recommendations over legally binding duties.[47] Advocates of WHO's non-legal approach claim that recommendations better serve public health objectives than binding rules because the undertaking of action depends on the willing cooperation of the sovereign state.[48] Soft law can be seen not only as a description of a type of norm but also as a process that seeks to build cooperation and consensus in achieving certain objectives.[49] WHO's soft law process on infectious diseases involves trying to persuade states to base decisions on rational epidemiological principles rather than rational or irrational fears about diseases or lost trade and tourist revenues. While attractive, this argument ignores the fact that recommendations and persuasion have not worked much better than binding rules in getting states to comply with the IHR.[50] The soft law process on infectious disease control has not been working well.

Other areas of international law touching on infectious disease control

Although the IHR and its predecessors constitute the main body of international legal rules on infectious disease control, other international legal subjects touch on the issue of infectious disease control. The many diverse factors behind EIDs illustrate that they are socio-economic problems of enormous complexity involving many sectors of a society and economy. In this part, I briefly highlight four major bodies of international law that fit into the EID discourse on the role of international law (Table 4.2).

Trade treaties designed to liberalize trade among states, like the General Agreement on Tariffs and Trade (GATT) and the North American Free Trade Agreement (NAFTA), often include provisions that allow the parties to restrict imports in order to protect animal, plant, or human life or health.[51] So-called sanitary and phytosanitary provisions represent the intersection of trade and public health agendas.[52] In many ways, international trade law attempts to balance trade and health as the IHR do. Under GATT, for example, import restrictions to protect human health are justified if they are necessary and do not represent arbitrary discrimination or a disguised restriction on trade (Article XX (b)).[53] The World Trade Organization (WTO) Agreement on the Application of Sanitary and Phytosanitary Measures imposes further disciplines on using trade restrictions to protect health.[54] The general thrust of this Agreement is to ensure that sanitary and phytosanitary measures are based on scientific principles so that health can be legitimately protected without hurting trade flows needlessly.[55] The IHR and trade treaties share the general interests of protecting populations against disease spread with minimal interference with world traffic.

The IHR and health provisions in trade treaties should not be seen, however, as complete mirror images. Trade treaties might be interpreted as giving states more discretion in imposing sanitary and phytosanitary measures than the IHR allows member states of WHO in response to

Table 4.2 Other areas of international law touching upon infectious disease control

Area of international law	Importance to infectious disease control
International trade law	Infectious diseases spread through international trade. Trade agreements usually allow products to be kept out of a state to protect health and under sanitary and phytosanitary provisions
International human rights law	The treatment of individuals who suffer from certain diseases, like HIV/AIDS, as well as access to public health services, have become matters addressed by international human rights law
International environmental law	Environmental degradation is a factor in the emergence and re-emergence of infectious diseases, making the efforts in international environmental law to protect the environment relevant for infectious disease control purposes
International arms control law	Experts are worried about increased likelihood that states and/or terrorist groups will use biological weapons, leading to efforts to strengthen international legal controls on biological weapons

disease outbreaks. For example, Peru suffered serious economic losses during its 1991 cholera epidemic because other states applied measures against Peruvian trade that were excessive under the IHR.[56] Some of the countries that imposed trade restrictions on Peru justified them under the GATT provisions allowing states to protect health.[57] Greater freedom to impose health-related trade restrictions under trade treaties than exists under the IHR might undermine the latter legal regime. The presence in trade treaties of dispute settlement and enforcement mechanisms can act, however, as a countervailing factor to any desire a state may have to use sanitary and phytosanitary measures as a protectionist device, depending on the effectiveness of such mechanisms.

Cogent arguments have been made that more coordination and cooperation between the WTO and WHO need to occur because their jurisdictions overlap in connection with infectious diseases.[58] Trade treaties might be an effective way to strengthen compliance with the IHR duty not to take excessive measures. For example, WHO plans in its revision of the IHR to state clearly what measures are excessive in responding to disease outbreaks in other states.[59] Trade treaties could bring pressure to bear on states to comply with such guidance from WHO by denying trade restrictive measures that exceed WHO guidelines any presumption of conformity with rules on health-related trade restrictions. Such cross-pollination of WHO and WTO legal regimes could strengthen both and improve international law on infectious disease control. At any rate, the volume and scope of the global food trade will ensure that international trade law remains very relevant to international efforts at infectious disease control.

International human rights law

Discrimination against persons suffering from AIDS during the 1980s by states in their immigration policies led to activists in public health and international law building a bridge between infectious disease control and international human rights law.[60] The building of this bridge also tied into WHO's work on a general human right to health.[61] Human rights law, therefore, relates to infectious disease control in two related ways.

First, the human rights discourse that developed in connection with anti-AIDS immigration policies suggested that national public health policies and interventions should be disciplined by respect for fundamental human rights.[62] In this suggestion can be seen the impact of the human rights revolution on public health strategies. The legal literature on AIDS in the United States during the 1980s discusses the need to update American public health law to integrate better with modern notions of civil rights and due process.[63] Plans to revamp existing international law on infectious disease control has to keep the human rights perspective in mind.

Second, the general human right to health focuses more on individual access to conditions and services necessary for health.[64] Adequate sanitation and water supplies are two important elements in achieving the public's health that do not exist in many developing countries today.[65] In addition, access to public health services has been deteriorating in the developed and developing worlds in recent decades.[66] It is not far-fetched to argue that the extent of the EID problem globally reflects the lack of progress on the part of states in fulfilling the human right to health. The gap between this right and reality challenges international law on infectious disease control in a different way. To create the conditions that would allow states to improve enjoyment of the right to health, international law has to be made to address *how* states provide public health, which is an issue not confronted by the IHR and its predecessors. The human right to health may also mean that developed states have to transfer financial resources to developing countries to help them improve public health conditions and services.[67] Such considerations dramatically expand the scope of an international legal regime on infectious disease control.

International environmental law

Experts often list environmental degradation as a factor behind the EID problem.[68] Such degradation can be very local, as illustrated by the evidence that deforestation brings humans into contact with new pathogens.[69] The environmental degradation may also be global, as illustrated by the fears that global warming will expand the geographical range of mosquitoes, which act as vectors for an assortment of infectious diseases, such as malaria and dengue fever.[70] Concern about environmental protection seems, therefore, to be important to international infectious disease control.

If such concern is warranted, then international environmental law becomes very relevant to infectious disease control. The success or failure of the treaty on global warming[71] can have direct consequences for international infectious disease control. As in the human rights context, the relevance of international environmental law to infectious disease control expands considerably the scope of an international legal regime on infectious disease control.

International controls on biological weapons

A theme in EID literature concerns the heightened awareness and worry about the production and use of biological weapons by states or terrorist groups.[72] Sometimes described as the 'poor man's atomic bomb', biological weapons represent a frightening threat to populations that are very vulnerable to the release of lethal pathogenic microbes. Although a multilateral treaty prohibits the development, production and stockpiling of biological weapons,[73] experts have questioned the effectiveness of this treaty.[74] In addition, the treaty does not deter terrorist groups from utilizing bioterrorism in their strategies.[75] States parties to the multilateral treaty on biological weapons completed in December 1996 their fourth review conference of the treaty by supporting work to draft a protocol to improve verification of compliance with the treaty to be concluded before 2001.[76] The international legal regime on infectious disease control has to include rules to address not only the threat from infectious diseases created by ordinary human activities but also the threat that pathogenic microbes might be intentionally used for malevolent purposes.

Current developments in the wake of the EID threat

The global nature of the EID threat reinforces the need for international law in creating strategies to deal with EIDs. In this section, I briefly describe some current developments in infectious disease diplomacy to shed some light on what roles international law may have in the era of EIDs (Table 4.3).

Multilateral initiatives

One of the most important developments is WHO's planned revision of the IHR. In December 1995 an informal WHO consultation group made recommendations on revising the IHR,[77] which recommendations WHO's new Division of Emerging and Other Communicable Diseases Surveillance and Control (EMC) is currently attempting to translate into substantive amendments to the IHR.[78] EMC estimates that the revised IHR will shortly be presented for approval by the World Health Assembly.[79] According to EMC, four principles are driving the IHR revision:

1. The current role and function of the IHR should be revised and expanded. The current practice of immediately reporting of only three specific diseases which should be replaced by the immediate reporting to WHO of defined syndromes representing disease occurrence of international importance and of all useful epidemiological information.

Table 4.3   Overview of some current developments in infectious disease control international law and diplomacy

Multilateral initiatives	Regional initiatives	Bilateral initiatives
1. WHO revision of the International Health Regulations	1. Group of Seven industrialized countries	1. US–European Union Transatlantic Agenda EID task force
2. Efforts of EMC division of WHO to carry out its strategic plan	2. Asia Pacific Economic Cooperation forum (APEC)	2. US–Japan Common Agenda
	3. European Community proposal for EC-wide surveillance and control network	3. US–Russia cooperation
		4. US–South Africa cooperation

2. The revised IHR should be accompanied by a practical handbook that defines the criteria for the requirements for international reporting and that otherwise facilitates the proper use of the IHR.
3. The revised IHR should be expanded to include a description of inappropriate or excessive interventions and should provide clear indications as to why these actions are not permitted.
4. The revised IHR should be integrated into all epidemic surveillance and control activities at global, regional and national level.[80]

Discourse about the proposed revisions is developing in the international legal literature; some analyses are critical of the revision proposals,[81] while others are more positive about the approach being adopted by EMC.[82] Of these principles, only the change from disease-specific reporting to syndrome reporting constitutes a substantive change from the prior IHR. Syndrome reporting would make the revised IHR applicable to a wider range of diseases than just cholera, plague and yellow fever. If the revisions follow the four principles listed above, the main set of international legal rules on infectious disease control will change from disease-specific reporting to syndrome reporting, which expands the scope of the duty to notify, but does little else to modify the framework established by the IHR and its predecessors.

For EMC, revision of the IHR constitutes only one aspect of its strategic plan to improve WHO's capabilities in the fight against EIDs. EMC has four strategic objectives: (1) strengthen global surveillance of infectious diseases (to which the revised IHR is intended to contribute); (2) strengthen national and international infrastructure necessary to deal with EIDs; (3) strengthen national and international capacity for the prevention and control of infectious diseases; and (4) support and promote research in infectious disease control.[83] In dedicating its 1996 World Health Report to the global crisis in infectious diseases,[84] WHO indicated that EIDs will form part of its multilateral responsibilities for promoting health for many years to come.

Regional initiatives

While WHO remains central to EID strategies, states are expanding their EID diplomacy to involve initiatives at the regional level as well. For example, both the Group of Seven industrialized nations and the participating states of the Asia Pacific Economic Cooperation (APEC) forum have acknowledged the importance of international cooperation on EIDs as part of their activities,[85] While such diplomatic acknowledgment does not create international law, it does indicate a level of seriousness about EIDs that cannot be overlooked. These diplomatic recognitions of EIDs help raise the issue of infectious disease control within regional frameworks previously concerned exclusively with other matters. The elevation of the EID problem may translate into regional agreements that will add to the body of international law on infectious disease control. Such diplomatic acknowledgments also constitute state practice specifically on EIDs that may eventually develop into customary international law.

A more extensive regional effort is underway in the European Community. The 1992 Treaty on European Union amended the Treaty of Rome to include a provision granting the European Commission limited powers in public health (Article 129).[86] The European Commission has drafted a proposal for the creation of a network for the epidemiological surveillance and control of infectious diseases in the European Community.[87] The Commission's proposal 'seeks to establish a system of close cooperation and effective coordination between Member States in the field of surveillance, both routine and emergency, with a view to improving the prevention and control in Europe of a certain number of serious communicable diseases which necessitate the introduction of measures for the protection of populations'.[88] If implemented, the proposal could begin to build a body of infectious disease control law for the European Community. European Health Ministers did not, however, greet the Commission's proposals with enthusiasm at their Council meeting in November 1996.[89] In contrast, the European Parliament offered amendments to the proposal on the grounds that the proposal did not go far enough to protect public health in the European Community.[90]

The tension apparently developing over the Commission's surveillance network proposal has not, however, developed to the acrimony exhibited in the controversy over 'mad cow disease' between Great Britain and the European Commission. This dispute took a legal turn in 1996 when the Commission imposed a worldwide ban on British beef exports, which in turn led to the British government challenging this ban before the European Court of Justice (ECJ). The ECJ held, among other things, that the Commission was justified in imposing the ban because such measure was taken to fulfill the Community objective of protecting public health.[91] This case establishes a precedent for the further development of infectious disease control law within the European Community.

Bilateral initiatives

Evidence of the growing importance of EID diplomacy comes in the form of the bilateral efforts that the United States has been making under its EID strategy. In 1996, EID working groups were established within the US–European Union Trans-Atlantic Agenda and the US–Japan Common Agenda.[92] These diplomatic agendas involve many issues, and the incorporation of EIDs into them indicates again how seriously some states are taking EIDs. The United States and the European Union have created an action plan for EIDs that includes (1) establishing a task force to develop and implement an effective global early-warning system and response network for infectious diseases; (2) increased training and professional exchanges on infectious diseases; (3) coordination of activities with WHO and other relevant international organizations; and (4) bilateral and multilateral cooperation on health-related matters (for example, AIDS and other infectious diseases).[93] In addition, EID cooperation efforts were launched between the United States and South Africa (under the Gore-Mbecki Commission) and Russia (under the Gore-Chernomyrdin Commission) during 1996.[94] While none of these bilateral initiatives by the United States can yet be considered substantive contributions to international law on infectious disease control, they contain the potential to evolve into bilateral agreements that would further develop international law on this topic.

What the future holds

Analysis of current developments in EID diplomacy offers a few clues about what the future holds for international law on infectious disease control. First, the multilevel nature of EID diplomacy suggests that states have decided not to rely solely on WHO to combat EIDs. Although revision of the IHR by WHO remains important, regional and bilateral initiatives also promise to begin to create international agreements and state practice on EID control and prevention. Activity at multiple levels of diplomacy could be interpreted as complementary to WHO's leadership or more skeptically, as an alternative to WHO-dominated initiatives.

Second, the bilateral and regional efforts under way, combined with the conservative nature of the IHR revision proposal, might mean that the innovative international legal developments will occur regionally and bilaterally. The time when a single multilateral legal instrument dominates international law on infectious disease control may be coming to an end.

Third, many of the regional and bilateral initiatives are happening between and among developed countries. Lurking in this positive development is the possibility of a two-tier system of international infectious disease control emerging. The top tier would be occupied by developed states that enjoy higher standards of public health and are moving towards greater cooperation through regional and bilateral EID projects. The bottom tier would be occupied by developing states that suffer from inadequate public health conditions and services and are left to rely on WHO. In addition, the history of international law on infectious disease control has always been tinged with a fear by developed states of disease importation from less affluent regions.[95] This fear has not disappeared and may encourage developed countries to band together first before facing the enormous problems in developing countries that contribute to the global EID threat. A two-tier international infectious disease control system would not, in some respects, be historically unique, as developed states enjoyed higher health standards than developing states during the twentieth century.[96] It is too early to predict the development of a two-tier system of international infectious disease control, and perhaps regional efforts within forums like the Pan-American Health Organization and APEC can create more North–South links in EID diplomacy. The warnings from public health experts about the global threat posed by EIDs make the possible uneven development of a global infectious disease control system worrisome because it is clear that the international community ignores at its peril the public health problems of the developing world at its peril.

Fourth, the intersections of infectious disease control and trade, human rights, environmental protection, and arms control promise to put EIDs on many international legal agendas. Such prominence should ensure that EIDs become a subject of international legal discourse for many years. The intersection between trade and infectious disease control may be particularly active as the WTO gathers momentum as the driving force in international trade. The number and complexity of the many intersections also pose the challenge of coordinating international law on infectious disease control with other substantive international legal regimes.

Conclusion

This chapter has undertaken a general review of the role of international law on the control of EIDs. The structure of the international system not only makes international law necessary to the control of infectious diseases but also subjects international law to limitations. The historical development of international law on infectious disease control underscores both the need for and limitations of international law in this area of international relations. Existing international law on infectious disease control has been exposed by the EID problem to be inadequate and ineffective, resembling soft law more than binding obligations. The unsatisfactory state of international law on infectious diseases becomes more daunting when the scope of the legal challenge expands to include many other substantive areas of international law. In response to the EID threat, WHO and states regionally and bilaterally are working to enhance the role of international law on the control of EIDs. Whether international law's role in infectious disease control improves because of the stimulus provided by EIDs remains to be seen. Ultimately it is important to remember that international law has no role beyond what states give it. It is, to paraphrase Edmund Burke, a mere instrument that quickly breaks down, absent obligations written in the heart.[97] Nations around the world seemingly recognize the threat EIDs pose to humanity. Whether this recognition reflects a superficial commitment to the EID problem or represents an obligation written in the heart to improve humanity's health will determine what role international law has in this new struggle against infectious diseases.

Acknowledgments

I wish to thank Peter Daniel DiPaloa and Jill M. Sears, research assistants, for their assistance during the preparation of this article, and Allyn L. Taylor, Bruce J. Plotkin, and Dr Stephen M. Ostroff for their helpful comments on an earlier draft of this chapter.

Notes

* International lawyers today interpret the phrase 'civilized nations' to mean states in the international system and do not intend in using this term to divide the world into civilized and uncivilized nations.

1 I. Brownlie, Statute of the International Court of Justice (1945), in *Basic Documents in International Law*, 4th edn (Oxford: Oxford University Press, 1995) p. 448.

2 I. Brownlie, *Principles of Public International Law*, 4th edn (Oxford: Oxford University Press, 1990).

3 Statute of the International Court of Justice, op. cit.

4 D. P. Fidler, 'Globalization, International Law, and Emerging Infectious Diseases', *Emerging Infectious Diseases*, 2 (1996a) pp. 77–84.

5 Ibid.

6 Ibid; D. P. Fidler, 'The Globalization of Public Health: Emerging Infectious Diseases and International Relations', *Indiana Journal of Global Legal Studies*, 5 (1997a).

7 U.S. Centers for Disease Control and Prevention, *Addressing Emerging Infectious Disease Threats: a Prevention Strategy for the United States* (Washington, DC: US Department of Health and Human Services, 1994); G. A. Gellert, A. K. Neumann and R. S. Gordon, 'The Obsolescence of Distinct Domestic and International Health Sectors', *Journal of Public Health Policy*, 10 (1989) pp. 421–4.

8   Fidler (1996a; 1997a), op. cit.
9   N. Howard-Jones, 'Origins of International Health Work', *British Medical Journal* (6 May 1950) pp. 1032–7.
10   Fidler (1996a), op. cit.
11   Howard-Jones, op. cit.
12   Ibid.
13   International Sanitary Convention (1903), in *Bevans*, 1 (1903) pp. 359–423.
14   World Health Organization, *International Health Regulations*, 3rd edn (Geneva: WHO, 1983).
15   Ibid.
16   World Health Organization, Division of Emerging and Other Communicable Diseases Surveillance and Control, *Emerging and Other Communicable Diseases Strategic Plan 1996–2000*, WHO/EMC/96.1 (Geneva: WHO, 1996).
17   D. P. Fidler, 'Challenging the Classical Concept of Custom: Perspectives on the Future of Customary International Law', *German Yearbook of International Law*, 39 (1996b) pp. 198–248.
18   S. Zamora, 'Is There Customary International Economic Law?' *German Yearbook of International Law*, 32, (1989) pp. 9–42; D. M. Bodansky, 'Customary (and Not So Customary) International Environmental Law', *Indiana Journal of Global Legal Studies*, 3 (1995) pp. 105–119.
19   Brownlie (1990), op. cit.
20   World Health Organization (1983), op. cit.
21   Ibid.
22   World Health Organization, *The International Response to Epidemics and Applications of the International Health Regulations: Report of a WHO Informal Consultant*, WHO/EMC/IHR/96.1 (Geneva: WHO, 1995); K. Tomasevski, 'Health' in O. Schacter and C. Joyner, *United Nations Legal Order* (Cambridge: Cambridge University Press, 1995); D. P. Fidler, 'Mission Impossible? International Law and Infectious Diseases', *Temple International Comparative Law Journal*, 10 (1996c) pp. 493–502; A. L. Taylor, 'Controlling the Global Spread of Infectious Diseases: Toward a Reinforced Role for the International Health Regulations', *Houston Law Review*, 32 (1997) pp. 1327–62; D. P. Fidler, 'Return of the Fourth Horseman: Emerging Infectious Diseases and International Law', *Minnesota Law. Review*, 81 (1997b) pp. 771–868.
23   Tomasevski, 'Health', op. cit.; P. J. Delon, *The International Health Regulations: A Practical Guide* (Geneva: WHO, 1975).
24   Taylor (1997), op. cit.; Fidler (1997b), op. cit.
25   L. Garrett, *The Coming Plague: Newly Emerging Diseases in a World Out of Balance* (New York: Penguin Books, 1994).
26   Fidler (1997b), op. cit.; L. Gordenker, 'The World Health Organization: Sectoral Leader or Occasional Benefactor?' in R. A. Coate (ed.) *U.S. Policy and the Future of the United Nations* (New York: Twentieth Century Fund Press, 1994) pp. 167–91.
27   Fidler (1996a), op. cit.
28   World Health Assembly (May 12, 1995), 'Revision and Updating of the International Health Regulations,' WHO Document WHA 48.7.
29   Fidler (1996b), op. cit.
30   Brownlie (1990), op. cit.
31   Fidler (1996b), op. cit.

32 Ibid.
33 Brownlie, op. cit.
34 Ibid.
35 Ibid.
36 Statute of the International Court of Justice, op. cit.
37 Brownlie (1990), op. cit.
38 Ibid.
39 Ibid; Statute of the International Court of Justice, op. cit.
40 World Health Organization (1983), op. cit.
41 Delon, op. cit.
42 E. Zoller, *Peacetime Unilateral Remedies: an Analysis of Countermeasures* (New York: Transnational Publishers, 1984).
43 Statute of the International Court of Justice, op. cit.; Brownlie, op. cit.
44 Fidler (1996c), op. cit.; Taylor, op. cit.; Fidler (1997b), op. cit.; B. J. Plotkin, 'Mission Possible: the Future of the International Health Regulations', *Temple International Comparative Law Journal*, 10 (1996) pp. 503–15; B. J. Plotkin and A. M. Kimball (1997), 'Designing the International Policy and Legal Framework for Emerging Infection Control: First Steps', *Emerging Infectious Diseases*, 3 (1997) 1–9.
45 W. M. Reisman, 'A Hard Look at Soft Law', *American Society of International Law Proceedings* (1988) pp. 371–7.
46 D. M. Leive, *International Regulatory Regimes: Case Studies in Health, Meteorology and Food* (Lexington, Mass.: Lexington Books, 1976).
47 A. L. Taylor, 'Making the World Health Organization Work: a Legal Framework for Universal Access to Conditions for Health', *American Journal of Legal Medicine*, 18 (1992) pp. 301–46.
48 C.-H. Vignes, 'The Future of International Health Law: WHO Perspectives', *International Digest of Health Legislation*, 40 (1989) pp. 16–19.
49 P. M. Dupuy (1991), 'Soft Law and the International Law of the Environment', *Michigan Journal of International Law*, 12 (1991) pp. 420–35.
50 Fidler (1997b), op. cit.
51 World Trade Organization (1993), *Agreement on the Application of Sanitary and Phytosanitary Measures*.
52 Plotkin and Kimball, op. cit.
53 General Agreement on Tariffs and Trade (1947), in J. H. Jackson, W. J. Davey and A. O. Sykes, Jr., *Documents Supplement to Legal Problems of International Economic Relations*, 3rd edn.
54 World Trade Organization (1993), op. cit.
55 Plotkin and Kimball, op. cit.
56 D. L. Heymann, 'The International Health Regulations: Ensuring Maximum Protection with Minimum Restriction', American Bar Association Program Materials on Law and Emerging and Re-Emerging Infectious Diseases, 5 August 1996, pp. 12–15.
57 GATT, *Analytical Index: Guide to GATT Law and Practice*, 6th edn (Geneva: GATT).
58 Plotkin and Kimball, op. cit.
59 World Health Organization (1995), op. cit.
60 Tomasevski, op. cit.
61 Taylor (1992), op. cit.

62   R. M. Jarvis, 'Advocacy for AIDS Victims: An International Law Approach', *University of Miami Inter-American Law Review*, 20 (1988) pp. 1–29.

63   L. Gostin, 'A Decade of a Maturing Epidemic: an Assessment and Directions for Future Public Policy', *American Journal of Legal Medicine*, 16 (1990) pp. 1–32.

64   Taylor (1992), op. cit.

65   L. Garrett, 'The Return of Infectious Disease', *Foreign Affairs*, 75, no.1 (1996) pp. 66–79.

66   Garrett (1994), op. cit.; National Science and Technology Council Committee on International Science, Engineering, and Technology Working Group on Emerging and Re-Emerging Infectious Diseases, *Infectious Diseases – a Global Health Threat* (Washington, DC: National Science and Technology Council, 1995).

67   Fidler (1996a), op. cit.; Fidler (1997b), op. cit.

68   S. S. Morse, 'Examining the Origins of Emerging Viruses', in S. Morse (ed.), *Emerging Viruses* (Oxford: Oxford University Press, 1993) pp. 10–28.

69   A. Gibbons, 'Where are "New" Diseases Born? Deforestation and Disease', *Science*, 261, pp. 680–1.

70   R. A. Kerr, 'Greenhouse Report Foresees Growing Global Stress', Science, 270 (1995) p. 731; J. A. Patz et al., 'Global Climate Change and Emerging Infectious Diseases', *Journal of the American Medical Association*, 275 (1996) pp. 217–23.

71   United Nations Framework Convention on Climate Change (1992), in *International Legal Materials*, 31, pp. 849–80.

72   U.S. Centers for Disease Control and Prevention (1994), op. cit.; Garrett (1996), op. cit.; National Science and Technology Council Committee, op. cit.

73   Convention on the Prohibition of the Development, Production, and Stockpiling of Bacteriological (Biological) and Toxin Weapons and Their Destruction (1972), in *United States Treaties*, 26, p. 583.

74   W. S. Carus, 'The Proliferation of Biological Weapons', in B. Roberts, *Biological Weapons: Weapons of the Future?'* (Washington, DC: Center for Strategic International Studies, 1993) pp. 19–27; J. F. Sopko, 'The Changing Proliferation Threat', *Foreign Policy*, Winter 1996–97, pp. 3–20.

75   M. J. Cetron and O. Davies,'The Future Face of Terrorism', *The Futurist*, 28 (1994) pp. 10–15.

76   Fourth Review Conference of the Parties to the Convention on the Prohibition of the Development, Production and Stockpiling of Bacteriological (Biological) and Toxin Weapons and on Their Destruction (1996), Final Declaration, BWC/CONF.IV/9.

77   World Health Organization (1995), op. cit.

78   World Health Organization (1996), op. cit.

79   Heymann, op. cit.

80   Ibid.

81   Fidler (1996c), op. cit.; Taylor (1997), op. cit.; Fidler (1997b), op. cit.

82   Plotkin, op. cit.; Heymann, op. cit.

83   World Health Organization (1996), op. cit.

84   World Health Organization, *The World Health Report 1996: Fighting Disease, Fostering Development* (Geneva: WHO, 1996).

85   National Science and Technology Council Committee, op. cit.; Group of Seven Industrialized Nations, 'Toward Greater Security and Stability in a More Cooperative World', 29 June 1996; personal correspondence from

S. M. Ostroff; Associate Director for Epidemiologic Science, National Centers for Disease Control, Atlanta: CDC, 21 November 1996.

86 Treaty Establishing the European Community (1992), in *European Union: Selected Instruments taken from the Treaties*, I, 265–6 (Brussels: European Community, 1995).

87 European Commission, 'Proposal for a European Parliament and Council Decision Creating a Network for the Epidemiological Surveillance and Control of Communicable Disease in the European Community', O. J. C123, 26 April 1996, pp. 10–13.

88 European Commission, 'Commission Communication Concerning Communicable Disease Surveillance Networks in the European Community', COM (96) 78, 7 March 1996.

89 Health Ministers Discuss Disease Network and EU Health Card, *European Report*, 16 November 1996.

90 'EP Modifies Proposals on a Network for Surveillance of Communicable Diseases and AIDS in Developing Countries', *Agence Europe*, 22 November 1996.

91 *United Kingdom* v. *E. C. Commission* (*Re*: Emergency Measures to Protect Against Bovine Spongiform Encephalopathy), Common Market Law Reports [1996] 3, pp. 1–21.

92 'Worldwide Network to Warn of Epidemics: Under Plan, U.S. and European Governments Will Take Lead in Reporting Outbreaks', *Washington Post*, 28 November 1996, A-9; and S. M. Ostroff, personal correspondence.

93 The New Transatlantic Agenda, available on the Internet at URL: http://europa.eu.int/en/agenda/tr06 ap2.html#ii7.

94 S. M. Ostroff, personal correspondence.

95 Howard-Jones, op. cit.; Fidler (1997b), op. cit.

96 Fidler, (1997a), op. cit.

97 E. Burke, 'First Letter on a Regicide Peace', in *The Writings and Speeches of Edmund Burke* (R. B. McDowell, ed.), IX, 187–264, (Oxford: Oxford University Press, 1995).

5

The Political Causes and Solutions of the Current Tuberculosis Epidemic

Kraig Klaudt

When presented with the facts of the tuberculosis epidemic for the first time, most people are profoundly puzzled. Something doesn't make sense. If highly effective anti-TB medicines are available, costing less than a few large bottles of aspirin for an entire course of treatment in some countries, why are nearly three million people still dying from TB each year? And, if the delivery system for these anti-TB medicines has been evaluated as being one of the most cost-effective health interventions for *any* disease, why is TB killing more youth and adults each year than AIDS, malaria, and all other infectious diseases combined? There is something clearly wrong with the equation.

The TB epidemic has vividly demonstrated that the best research developments and the most effective and affordable medical tools are irrelevant to public health if the political will and community resources to utilize them do not exist. Those who eagerly await breakthroughs for AIDS, cancer, heart disease and other diseases are advised to take note. There is little reason to expect that when life-saving scientific discoveries are made, these medicines or vaccines will be available – without political struggle – for the majority of people at risk from these diseases.

If the global tuberculosis epidemic is to be reduced substantially in the next ten years, it will be because eye-opening discoveries concerning the disease will be made in parliaments, congresses, ministries and boardrooms, rather than in the laboratories of research scientists. If funding and policy decisions are immediately taken to use existing medicines and tools more widely, the lives of millions of patients can be saved in the next few years. Hence, the creation of political will to address the TB epidemic has become an essential – if sometimes controversial – cornerstone of the World Health Organization's Global TB Programme efforts to reverse the epidemic.

The social transformation of TB in the twentieth century

In the mid-nineteenth century, tuberculosis brought about the death of nearly one in every seven people in Britain and was probably the single biggest killer of Europeans and North Americans. At that time, TB was arguably a disease even more pervasive and frightening than the current AIDS epidemic. Not only was TB incurable, but it also spread through the air. No change of behavior – short of holding one's breath indefinitely – could provide protection.

By the beginning of the twentieth century, TB case rates were on a gradual decline as social conditions improved in Europe and North America. Sanitaria may have also contributed to this decline by isolating infectious cases from the community. The discovery of a number of effective anti-TB medicines beginning in 1944 provided humanity the means to shut the door on the epidemic. In Europe and North America, these medicines were provided to most TB patients in sanitaria or hospitals in courses lasting a year or more, so it was relatively easy to ensure that patients took their treatment each day and were eventually cured. In wealthy countries, the number of annual TB cases and deaths declined steadily.

By the early 1980s, health officials in America were optimistic about the eventual eradication of the disease within their borders. In 1989, the US Department of Health and Human Services published 'A Strategic Plan for the Elimination of Tuberculosis in the United States', with a target date of 2010.[1] Even in Pakistan, a country with one of the worst TB situations in the world, with more than 200 000 cases a year, a leading anti-poverty association presented a medal to a key health official for his role in *eradicating* TB from the country.[2] At least four unforeseen developments[3] made a mockery of these premature epitaphs.

First, while tuberculosis cases were declining in wealthy countries, the epidemic was going largely unaddressed in developing countries.[4] The TB control strategy so effective for wealthy countries was unfeasible in countries lacking the hospital infrastructure and operating funds to ensure that medicines would be taken without interruption for the entire course of treatment. Attempts to provide out-patient TB treatment often accomplished more harm than good in developing countries. Unsupervised patients would take enough medicines to feel better and then discontinue treatment, only to relapse and continue to infect others. Rather than dying from tuberculosis, these patients were provided with enough medicine to survive, but not enough to prevent them from infecting a dozen other people each year.

Second, there was – and continues to be – much naivety among wealthy countries concerning the degree to which domestic public health measures can provide immunity from global epidemics. With increased travel (airlines now transport over a billion passengers each year), migration and immigration, a seemingly exotic outbreak in Kinshasa one week has the potential to become a crisis in Kansas City the next. In Scandinavian countries, nearly half of new TB cases can be traced to travelers and foreign-born individuals; in the United States, France and Germany the percentage is close to one-third. Still, most industrialized countries focus their public health resources on prevention efforts among their domestic population, as if human-made borders can magically ward off germs and viruses. This perspective can be seen in a 1993 report by the US Office of Technology Assessment:

> A potential danger of increasing United States support of TB efforts abroad is that it might divert resources from domestic TB control activities. The Federal Government has already laid out an ambitious domestic agenda to control TB for which there may not be sufficient funds to fully implement in the short-run. If money for expanded TB control efforts outside the United States would come from appropriations that would otherwise go to domestic public health and research activities, Congress may need to weigh the value of supporting efforts abroad against the impact that money would have on the health of people with TB at home.[5]

In 1997, the United States spent nearly a billion dollars to maintain a highly developed TB control program for treating approximately 22 000 new cases, but provided only $2 million in foreign aid to less-developed countries to help them control their severely worsening TB crises. While sustaining a strong domestic TB control program is certainly in the best interests of the American public, so is addressing the international TB crisis. Recent census data show that one in ten American citizens are of foreign birth. Five of the six leading countries of origin for immigrants to the United States – Mexico, the Philippines, China, India and Vietnam – are home to some of the most serious tuberculosis problems in the world.

A third factor accelerating TB's return has been the HIV/AIDS epidemic. Twenty years ago, few epidemiologists would have anticipated the advent of a virus that would so quickly and thoroughly destroy the immune system and unleash latent TB infections. Yet, this is exactly what HIV accomplishes in those who carry the TB bacilli in their lungs. Currently, about 10 percent of all new TB cases can be attributed to HIV causing TB infection to rapidly progress to sickness. Africa has experienced the greatest impact of the dual epidemic. In Zambia and Malawi, for example, HIV has caused the number of annual TB cases to increase fourfold in the span of ten years.[6]

And finally, the world was unprepared for an increase in sudden, often uncontainable outbreaks of multidrug-resistant TB (MDR TB). MDR TB is a human-made phenomenon resulting from erratic delivery of drug supplies, unsupervised administration of anti-TB medicines or medical incompetence. Incomplete and infrequent intake of medicines provides an opportunity for naturally-resistant TB bacilli to replicate. MDR TB is threatening to change the rules for curing TB patients. While the drugs to cure TB cost little more than $30 or $40 in most resource-poor countries, the cost of treating multidrug-resistant TB rises to at least $7000 per patient in low-income countries and around $180 000 in wealthy countries, with little guarantee that the patient will be cured.[7] Recent studies have documented that these TB 'superbugs' are far from isolated occurrences; some regions of the world are now reporting multidrug-resistance in over 20 percent of their TB cases.[8]

While these four factors were converging in the mid-1980s to fuel the TB epidemic, public awareness and political support for TB control was drifting in the opposite direction. From the beginning of the twentieth century until the present day, tuberculosis evolved from being Europe and North America's most feared and talked-about disease to a low public health priority overshadowed by the threat of AIDS and other newly emerging diseases. Public attention that had once been preoccupied with the consumption of Franz Kafka, Thomas Mann and George Orwell became focused on the immune status of Rock Hudson, Liberace, and Magic Johnson. Activist TB patient organizations and creative postage stamp campaigns which thrived at the beginning of the century disbanded and were forgotten by the time ACT UP and AIDS quilts arrived toward the century's end. Yet, paradoxically, throughout the decline in social and political interest in the disease, tuberculosis was actually becoming epidemiologically and bacteriologically more formidable. Precisely because of society's neglect, TB was killing more people worldwide annually by the last decade of the twentieth century than during its first decade.

Symptoms of neglect

There is no lack of institutions to blame for allowing tuberculosis to disappear from the agendas of policy-makers during the 1970s and 80s. Organizations entrusted to protect the public's health were increasingly forced to operate with reduced budgets during a period increasingly hostile to social programs, public health initiatives and foreign aid. With new demands on these institutions, funding for tuberculosis control was an easy target.

When WHO, the World Bank and the United Nations Development Programme established the Special Programme for Research and Training in Tropical Disease (TDR) in 1975, tuberculosis was not included among the research initiative's six diseases. By 1988, the World Health Organization had only one medical officer responsible for tuberculosis monitoring and control at its Geneva headquarters. Four decades earlier, WHO had nearly 50 medical staff assigned to address TB in its European regional office alone.

Bilateral aid for TB control was being disbursed at similarly embarrassing levels. In 1990, only $16 million in bilateral and multilateral support was being provided by donors to support the TB control efforts of developing countries. This represented approximately 0.03 percent of the nearly $50 billion of foreign aid disbursed that year.

Support for TB control services was dramatically reduced in many wealthy countries. Funding for TB control for the Centers for Disease Control and Prevention and most state and local health budgets in the United States were all but eliminated by 1970.[9] New York City's TB control budget decreased from $40 million in 1968 to only $4 million in 1988. In 1986, the British government disbanded the tuberculosis unit of its Medical Research Council, which had played a significant role in previous decades in investigating means of controlling the TB epidemic in developing countries.

Support for TB control in endemic countries also remained low, but for very different reasons. Previous TB control initiatives which had relied on BCG vaccinations and self-administered treatment were unsuccessful and resulted in much fatalism about the prospects of controlling the disease. Death from TB became accepted as an unfortunate inevitability for the poorest and disenfranchised segments of society. In India, outlays on tuberculosis represented only 1 percent of the country's health budget during the period from 1992 to 1997. Though TB is the leading infectious killer of youth and adults in India (one million cases in 1996), TB control allocations were just ahead of what was spent on

Guinea worm eradication (nine cases in 1996).[10] Health sector resource allocations in other developing countries have been even more askew. It is not uncommon to find the majority of a Ministry of Health's resources in some low-income countries spent on expensive medical gadgetry and surgeries to preserve the longevity of wealthy members of society, rather than on primary health care and basic, cost-effective interventions to help protect the lives of most citizens. According to one doctor, 'Instead of investing in the transport required for a rural tuberculosis service, countries buy equipment for expensive operating theatres where there is no surgeon.'[11]

In recent decades, support for TB control among NGOs was limited to a number of small TB and lung associations. In Europe and North America, many of these had all but abandoned tuberculosis to focus on other chest diseases and to discourage the use of tobacco. The American Lung Association, for example, began as the National Association for the Study and Prevention of Tuberculosis in 1904 but gradually reduced its involvement in the international TB epidemic.[12] Exceptionally, only a few TB NGOs remained primarily focused on tuberculosis, resisting the temptation to redirect their efforts to other lung diseases. The Royal Netherlands Tuberculosis Association (KNCV), the Paris-based International Union Against TB and Lung Disease (IUATLD) and the National Public Health Association in Norway were perhaps the only international organizations to make progress against the global TB epidemic in the 1980s. In countries such as Tanzania, Malawi, Benin, Mozambique and Nicaragua, the IUATLD pioneered the development and testing of the effective strategy now known as DOTS (Directly Observed Treatment, Short-course).

TB has also been a less-than-exciting area for ambitious medical staff to enter compared with AIDS or other newly emerging infectious diseases. Discussion on tuberculosis was all but absent in the education of North American and European medical students in the 1980s. By one account, some medical schools were devoting less than two hours to TB, with students in one school being told to skip the pages devoted to TB in their medical textbooks.[13]

Finally, support for TB research efforts had also come to a virtual standstill. The last of the ten drugs now available against TB – rifampicin – was approved in 1966. In subsequent years, the pharmaceutical industry virtually abandoned the testing of compounds for additional anti-TB medicines. Research into TB was, in part, resurrected in the late 1980s with the arrival of AIDS, but this was initially due to a concern about AIDS rather than TB. Nearly a third of scientific journal articles on TB in this decade have focused on aspects of TB/HIV co-infection.

Hindsight has near-perfect vision. One would not expect health officials to so quickly and drastically reduce their efforts to fight an airborne disease which had afflicted humanity for thousands of years, especially with a reservoir of two billion people still infected with the bacteria. However, the demise or survival of social initiatives is ultimately decided by political assessments based on *who* is perceived to be affected.

Factors contributing to low prioritization of TB in the 1980s

There may be a number of reasons why TB control has been a low priority in recent decades. A century-long decline in TB rates in industrialized countries likely encouraged a false sense of security. Closure of TB sanitaria created the public perception that TB was no longer a serious problem. Even when TB cases began increasing in industrialized countries, overconfidence in the powers of science and modern medicine may have caused some denial that humanity had failed to conquer the disease. The advent of AIDS also increasingly commanded the attention of health policy makers.

Yet, the most convincing explanation for neglect of the TB epidemic is found not in the arena of public health or medicine, but of social injustice. Segments of society holding wealth and power believed they had been spared from the mortal threat of tuberculosis and were relatively unmotivated to address the impact of the epidemic on those living in poverty. Governments which had virtually eliminated the disease within their own borders were unmoved by the devastation the epidemic was causing in resource-poor countries. Unfortunate choices were made by government officials to utilize power and allocate resources in support of initiatives having far less cost-effective benefits in protecting the health and survival of the public. Institutions which influence the political process – NGOs, associations, foundations and the media – frequently mirrored this apathy for the health and survival of tuberculosis patients.

For the middle class and elite of resource-rich countries, TB increasingly came to be seen as an exotic, distant threat that affected 'them' and not 'us'. TB became a disease of the faceless masses in far away lands, rather than the affliction of one's next-door neighbor. Television, which has the potential to globalize our view of the world, has been more successful at personalizing our outlook. Primetime presentations of human dramas – from celebrity murder trials to the sexual affairs of politicians – increasingly serve as the furnace in which modern Western values are forged. Accordingly, the majority of Americans have come to care more about whether or not a Michigan child receives a donated kidney, than worrying whether or not any progress is being made to save 30 million people in far away lands who may die in the next decade from TB. The author of a letter to the editor of the *Glasgow Herald* in the United Kingdom decries these priorities:

A million women die in childbirth every year: this is a tragedy. Thirty-five thousand children under age five die every day of preventable diseases: this is a tragedy. Three million people die each year of tuberculosis: this is a tragedy.

A single sperm whale died in the Firth of Forth earlier this year: this is not, by any stretch of the imagination, a tragedy (your headline, July 2).[14]

In many ways, the return of TB parallels the early years of the AIDS epidemic. Initially, in North America AIDS was seen only to affect marginalized segments of society, such as homosexuals, IV drug users, prostitutes and Haitians. Consequently, government funding, research and media coverage was not forthcoming. Only when AIDS was seen to be affecting heterosexuals, celebrities, children and other purported 'innocent victims' did the disease begin to command political attention. Similarly, if the TB epidemic had not begun to increase in industrialized countries and threaten to again become incurable for middle and upper-class citizens, it is unlikely that support for controlling the disease would have reemerged. According to one journalist who has frequently reported on efforts to control TB:

Scores of homeless African Americans and Hispanics had died in the USA from incurable TB before newspaper editors took interest. It took the death of a white prison guard at Syracuse to catapult the issue onto the front page of the *New York Times*. Similarly in the UK, it would usually require the fillip of an unexpected location like a Scottish public school or an English opera house for an outbreak of the disease to rise up the news and feature schedules.[15]

Forces of social injustice and neglect were abetted by four other significant factors which contributed to TB becoming a low political priority: lack of epidemiological and economic data on the epidemic; lack of clarity about the solution; lack of media coverage; and absence of leadership.

Lack of Epidemiological Data and Economic Analysis

The priorities of medical investigation in wealthy countries underwent a significant change during the 1970s and 80s. In many countries, public health infrastructures and surveillance systems – which had previously served as an early warning system for outbreaks of infectious diseases – were dismantled. In the United States, for example, medical investigations increasingly focused on consumer protection issues. Vaccines were, after all, proving effective against smallpox and other infectious diseases, while nearly every product and additive was suspected of causing cancer, birth defects or heart disease.

The world is still recovering from the blows dealt to the public health infrastructure during this period. The money saved by cutting corners on TB treatment services has failed to collect interest over the years. Rather, these 'cost-saving' measures have contributed to the undetected emergence of drug-resistant strains years later which come with a $100 000-plus price tag for treatment. Lack of surveillance has also made it difficult to document the necessity for higher prioritization of different health interventions. For many years, TB control has been a low funding priority, in part because funds to investigate the extent of the problem were limited, and vice versa.

Lack of clarity about the solution

As recently as 1995, tuberculosis control faced a serious marketing challenge. Nobody – including TB control professionals themselves – could clearly and quickly articulate the means for controlling the epidemic. The highly effective TB control strategy developed by Dr Karel Styblo went by obscure technical titles such as 'The Framework for TB Control', or 'The Styblo Method'. As a result, the most recognizable TB intervention for the majority of policy-makers continued to be the much-limited BCG vaccination, which has little effect in preventing the disease in adults.

Even worse, the vast majority of communications and promotion strategies surrounding tuberculosis were failing to target the most crucial audiences. Communications and media strategies used to promote the control of TB were usually IEC (Information, Education and Communication) campaigns, an approach commonly used with other diseases such as breast-feeding, sanitation and AIDS prevention.[16] Most TB control promotional efforts in endemic countries prematurely focused on the education and compliance of the patient, when the compliance of health workers and the support of policy-makers was actually more essential to the control of TB. Patients were being assured that if they took their medicines, they would be cured, when in fact frequent interruptions in drug supplies, confusion about proper drug regimens, misdiagnosis and lack of adequate laboratories sabotaged the patient's best efforts.

Not media friendly

It has been observed that if an issue does not exist in the media, it also fails to exist in politics. This maxim goes a long way towards explaining why TB control has been a low political priority, as it is difficult to imagine a more media-repellent affliction. TB is the oldest infectious disease known to humanity – found in mummies from ancient Egypt – so there is nothing new about the disease. As a slow-moving infection, it provides few opportunities for breaking CNN reports. The TB epidemic is not particularly camera-friendly either, as it causes the lungs to slowly deteriorate invisibly inside the body over a period of years. In short, the TB bacillus lacks all the newsworthiness exhibited by a new, exotic disease such as Ebola which can quickly and dramatically bleed its victims to death.

Compounding these limitations, TB has so far lacked the involvement of celebrities which has helped attract attention to other diseases. Currently, there are no Jerry Lewis Labor Day Telethons to raise money for TB drugs and supplies. Unlike AIDS and cancer, there have yet to be any prime-time death watches for rock stars, actors, designers and athletes suffering from TB.[17] Not that TB has failed to afflict the rich and famous; but society's elite are able to afford treatment and usually prefer to be quietly cured. As one health official cynically put it, 'the best thing that could happen for the millions of TB patients around the world would be for one famous Hollywood actress to catch multidrug-resistant TB.'

Lack of leadership

In most instances, campaigns to address important social issues are only as powerful as their political leaders. The fact that James Grant provided dynamic vision for child survival strategies and Jimmy Carter has championed the prevention of river blindness and Guinea worm disease has made all the difference in progressing against these challenges. For tuberculosis, however, such political leadership has been missing. In fact, public figures who have been personally involved with tuberculosis have even been reluctant to fight for its control. Dr Halfdan Mahler, a former TB physician who spent over a decade fighting the disease in Ecuador and India, served as WHO's director general from 1973 to 1988, a period during which WHO's TB surveillance and control capacity was dismantled. Nelson Mandela, who contracted TB on Robben Island in 1988, has not yet fully addressed his country's TB crisis, believed by many to be the worst in the world. Mohammed Ali Jinnah, the first governor of Pakistan, hid his bout with the disease, and his country remains in a state of denial about the seriousness of the problem. Throughout her life, Mother Theresa was publicly silent about her own TB illness, even while ministering care to countless numbers of TB patients. With high-profile leaders unwilling to make an issue out of the TB epidemic, it is not surprising that dynamic leadership in support of TB control has been equally absent in Ministries of Health, medical schools, research institutions and national TB programs.

In a similar way, tuberculosis specialists and chest physicians have frequently become their own worst enemies in building political support for TB control. These doctors and researchers often seem desensitized by the magnitude of an epidemic that produces millions of cases and billions of infections. Even when there are thousands of people infected with multidrug-resistant TB in a country, TB control officials will often present these numbers with no sense of urgency. Three percent multidrug-resistant levels are dismissed by some national TB programs as being low and acceptable (in Thailand, for example, that would represent over a thousand MDR TB cases). Meanwhile, governments are being rallied to take all sorts of extreme actions for threats which cause less mortality, such as an outbreak of the plague in India that may have affected 200 people; an outbreak of Ebola killing 200, or BSE which may have affected a dozen or more people.

The willingness to do something different

In 1989, the World Health Organization had only a small unit with an annual budget of around $500 000 to help lead the world's response to the global TB crisis. Like most United Nations entities, this unit was being called on to be all things to all countries and constituencies. With the appointment of a new unit chief, it was determined that if progress was going to be made against tuberculosis, some risks would need to be taken.

The TB Unit decided to focus its efforts on just a few countries to assist their TB control efforts, analyze the results, and learn from the mistakes. In 1989, Dr Styblo accompanied WHO staff to Tanzania and Malawi to introduce them to his strategy for controlling TB. In Tanzania during the 1980s, Styblo had developed a treatment system of checks and balances that provided high cure rates at a cost affordable for most developing countries. It was then tested in countries such as Malawi, Nicaragua and Mozambique, demonstrating that it would work even in the midst of extreme poverty and civil war. However, this new system had not been adopted by most other countries. In 1991, less than one percent of the world's TB patients were being treated through Styblo's effective system.

The challenge was to take recent innovations in TB control made by Styblo and the International Union Against TB & Lung Disease and craft the most essential elements into a technical package that could be used in any country. Styblo's system involved nearly 700 different tasks, but after careful study in Malawi and Tanzania, WHO determined that fewer than 100 were essential to run a successful TB control program. These tasks were subsequently explained in new WHO treatment guidelines and training modules applicable for any country.

Separately, the Chinese Ministry of Health had invited the World Bank to design a project to help deal with its extensive TB epidemic. Tuberculosis was then killing 400 000 people a year and was expected to worsen, due to the economic pressures placed on the health system as China's economy liberalized away from central planning. In July 1990, the World Bank invited Styblo to help design a TB control project for China. With the help of WHO, Styblo refined the approach he had developed in Africa so that it would suit China's health system. With World Bank funding and technical support from the World Health Organization, a pilot project was launched among two million people in five pilot counties of Hebei Province, near Beijing. By the end of 1991, this pilot project was achieving phenomenal results, more than doubling cure rates and eventually achieving 94 percent cure rates. This provided the basis for a larger World Bank project covering half of the country.

By late 1991, it was becoming clear that, in spite of initial successes in Africa and China, there was still little interest by most governments and donor agencies in using this effective strategy to attack TB. That winter, during a pivotal meeting of public health experts in Boston, three important developments took place. First, WHO's TB Unit committed a large share of its resources to enable Dr Chris Murray of the Harvard School of Public Health to measure the cost-effectiveness of Styblo's TB control approach. This research would later provide the basis for the analysis of TB in the World Bank's 1993 *World Development Report*. Second, the World Bank began discussing the possibility of reassigning key staff from its China TB control project to assist WHO in replicating these efforts. And third, TB Unit staff reached the conclusion that it would accomplish more by promoting the widespread use of existing, effective tools, rather than by making the development of new tools its top priority.

The next important step was taken a year later. At the Unit's Technical Research and Coordination advisory body meeting, the lack of political interest in controlling the TB epidemic was frankly discussed. Dr Dixie Snider, veteran of many public health campaigns with the Centers for Disease Control and Prevention in the United States, kept steering discussions back to the same common obstacle: the lack of political will to control TB. He summarized the situation when he observed, 'If we keep on doing the same old thing, we'll keep on getting the same old results.' Eventually, the group came around to concluding that they had been placing all of their hopes on using medical and research initiatives to address what was essentially a political challenge. By the end of the meeting, the committee recommended that advocacy and public awareness become a central component of the Unit's efforts, declaring that 'the most important activity to be undertaken is strong advocacy for increased support of the Tuberculosis Programme'. Within a few months, the TB Unit recruited an advocacy specialist and contracted the services of a political consulting firm to initiate a new approach to fighting the TB epidemic.

The subsequent TB advocacy efforts which began early in 1993 have sometimes been controversial within the World Health Organization. While WHO has a mandate to be both a normative technical body and an advocate for health, it has historically been more comfortable with the former role rather than the latter. Within this internal organizational context, the newly-elevated Global TB Programme began to utilize a number of advocacy strategies to help generate political support for controlling TB. These strategies included personally involving non-TB control experts; encouraging analytical comparison of costs and benefits to force priority setting; and empowering NGOs as TB control advocates. However, three strategies – above and beyond all others – proved essential in helping to make TB control a higher political priority. First, documenting the extent of the problem so that it would be relevant to policy-makers. Second, packaging and presenting the solution so it would appeal to policy-makers. And third, utilizing the media to encourage decision-makers to take action.

Documenting the Problem

Policy makers – and those who influence them – have little interest in the technical details of any proposal. They must be persuaded that an initiative fits into their agenda, makes economic sense, and that dire consequences will be faced if no action is taken. Above all, they must be convinced that the issue is of immediate relevance to their own constituency.

Building a case for TB control was no small challenge, given the apathy which surrounded the disease. Fortunately, through the dedicated efforts of WHO's TB Programme and Chris Murray, information was compiled in the early part the 1990s which conclusively demonstrated that TB had become the premier cause of mortality among youth and adults in developing countries. While the numbers from the exercises of WHO and Murray varied to some degree, the essential facts of the situation remained the same: rather than going away, the global TB epidemic was actually becoming more formidable than ever before. Moreover, the epidemic was primarily affecting the most economically productive age group – between the ages of 15 and 44.

The preparation of the World Bank's 1993 *World Development Report: Investing in Health* represented a watershed opportunity to document another aspect of the epidemic. The report presented unprecedented analysis on the cost-effectiveness of interventions to control different diseases and persuasively demonstrated that TB is one of the most cost-effective of all adult diseases to treat. For example, the medicines for an entire course of treatment in China now cost only $11 per patient, and usually between $30 to $40 in most developing countries. The entire cost of curing a TB patient with the DOTS strategy in developing countries – including staff and program costs – is usually around $200 a patient. This ranks TB control along with child vaccinations and oral rehydration as one of the most cost-effective health interventions.

As part of the preparation for the *World Development Report*, Murray also compiled information on foreign aid contributions toward various health interventions. This information showed that infectious diseases were sorely overlooked in health sector spending and that tuberculosis had become the most overlooked member of this neglected family. Infectious diseases accounted for nearly a third of all deaths in developing countries but receive less than two percent of all development assistance, with tuberculosis near the bottom of the list. The $811 million in foreign aid that was spent in 1990 on all infectious diseases is less that what some cities spend to construct, equip and staff one modern hospital.

The groundwork for effective political advocacy was now in place. The leading killer of youth and adults, and one of the most cost-effective diseases to control, was also one of the lowest priorities for health spending by aid agencies. If facts spoke for themselves in the world of resource allocations and policy decisions, little more would be needed. But in reality, additional motivation would be necessary to encourage rational decision-making. To begin with, policy-makers in donor countries had to be persuaded that this enormous global crisis also affected their own citizens. Fortunately for global TB control efforts, this case was becoming increasingly easy to make.

By 1990, it had become clear that the tuberculosis epidemic was returning to wealthy countries. From 1985 to 1992, TB cases increased in the United States by nearly 20 percent. During the last years of the 1980s, TB cases were also increasing in Austria, Denmark, Ireland, Italy, The Netherlands, Norway and Spain. In 1994, the World Health Organization reported that the number of annual TB cases had either stopped declining or had begun increasing in 20 of 27 Eastern European and former Soviet Union countries. In Russia in particular, the number of annual reported TB cases increased by nearly 70 percent over a period of just a few years.

New York City provides one example of the importance epidemiology has played in political advocacy for TB. In April 1991, the New York City Bureau of Tuberculosis Control conducted a systematic study on drug resistance in the city, which documented that the problem had reached dramatic proportions. Nearly 20 percent of New York City's TB cases were found to have multidrug-resistant TB. According to Dr Thomas Frieden, director of the Bureau of TB Control at the time, 'This study was essential in gaining medical credibility, priority within the Department of Health, media coverage, and funding.'[18] As these data were publicized, funding for US TB control efforts increased more than tenfold. In New York City alone, $40 million was made available for TB control in 1993.

Packaging and presenting the solution

As recently as 1995, the best strategy for addressing the worsening TB epidemic was unclear, even among TB control specialists. The delivery system for controlling TB in developing countries developed by Styblo had been standardized by WHO into a flexible package that could be utilized by any country. The result was a technical masterpiece, but a marketing nightmare. The 'Framework for TB Control', as it was originally called, consisted of five elements and nine key operations. It contained no new wonder drug or vaccine, but a series of uninspiring management and monitoring innovations. It was a product destined to sit on the shelf because – quite simply – it lacked a memorable name and image to which non-specialists could relate.

In 1995, the name for this strategy was born upon noticing that the word 'STOP' on a draft cover of an upcoming Global TB Programme publication resembled – upside down – one of the central elements of the Framework for TB Control; that being 'DOT' or directly observed therapy. It just needed an 'S'. With small modifications to emphasize that a specific combination of TB medicines, known as *short-course chemotherapy*, should be used, and that patients should be provided with comprehensive *treatment* to ensure they are documented as being cured, the product name for effective TB control, Directly Observed Treatment, Short-course, or 'DOTS' was created.

Of the five essential elements in the DOTS strategy, it was decided to emphasize the supportive bond between the patient and the health worker, who watches to ensure that each dose of medicines is taken. This low-tech, person-centered element has proved to be the most memorable feature of the DOTS strategy. By creating a structure which ensures that health workers are accountable to watch patients take each dose of anti-TB medicines and monitor their progress, it is possible to double cure rates for TB patients in most developing countries.

In the first year after introduction, DOTS was greeted with enthusiasm in most quarters, *except* among TB control professionals. With the exception of Styblo himself, most TB specialists resented what they believed to be the simplification and popularization of a complex and multifaceted strategy. Yet use of this TB control strategy has multiplied many-fold since 1995, again demonstrating the important role communication and marketing play in advancing public health measures.

Those trained in medicine frequently assume that facts will 'speak for themselves', even in a political context. Yet, these same authorities are often found lamenting how unreceptive policy-makers can be toward addressing urgent health issues. Often, it is not recognized that an investment in the packaging and presentation of one's initiative is as essential as funding its research and development. Strategies to change society's sexual behavior or to establish a cold chain for childhood vaccination campaigns are complex technical undertakings which have taken years of research to develop. However, political and public support for these interventions has materialized by marketing them through simple, obvious concepts and symbols. A condom, for example, has come to represent the means of controlling AIDS, though a condom is quite useless without accompanying education, social marketing and distribution strategies. The few seconds it takes to vaccinate a child is only the most visible element of a lengthy and multifaceted strategy for child survival. Likewise, the Global TB Programme's investment in the marketing of DOTS has helped focus policy makers on the most essential TB control practices, before providing them with all the potentially mind-numbing details.

The presentation of health issues to policy-makers represents an additional challenge. Few officials have time to stay informed on developments pertaining to their own disciplines, much less digest the avalanche of other information which reaches their desks each day. Most people will not pay attention to a new, seemingly peripheral issue unless they are surprised, shocked or entertained in its presentation. Recognizing this quandary, the Global TB Programme has adapted a distinctly unbureaucratic communications style in order to help capture the attention of key audiences. By presenting much of its advocacy information through the creative use of comic books, interactive reports, dramatic photographs and vivid illustrations, the Programme helps ensure that, not only will its materials be noticed by target audiences, but core messages will also be remembered.[19]

Utilizing the media

Media relations on neglected social issues is not for the faint of heart. Nor is it particularly well-suited for clinicians who have been conditioned throughout their medical training to speak in precise technical terms, qualify every assertion and resist simplification. Yet it has been precisely because key physicians have been willing to speak in soundbites and make controversial statements that tuberculosis has begun to return to the public's agenda.

Since 1992, media coverage of TB has nearly quadrupled in leading international media outlets.[20] Four Americans, Dr Dixie Snider, Dr Thomas Frieden, Dr Lee Reichman and Dr Barry Bloom led the way by calling attention to outbreaks of MDR TB in New York City and to the worsening global situation. In 1993 during a special meeting in London, the World Health Organization took the unprecedented step of declaring a 'global TB emergency'. That phrase, coined by Peter Schechter of Clopeck, Leonard & Schechter, was pivotal to helping the launch of the Global TB Programme's advocacy efforts. Health slogans have come and gone, but fortunately this particular slogan managed to avoid a lengthy deliberation which surely would have resulted in a warning of a 'tuberculosis problem almost everywhere'.

The challenge has been to sustain media attention year after year in order to build a solid foundation for long-term political commitment. The Global TB Programme has succeeded by drawing new media attention to what should be old, obvious facts about the epidemic. International headlines have appeared highlighting that 'India is Sitting on a TB Timebomb', 'South Africa's TB Crisis is the Worst in the World', 'TB Killing More People Now Than At Any Other Time In History' and 'DOTS is the Biggest Health Breakthrough of the 1990s'. One of the dubious advantages of TB's neglect, it seems, is that information about its severity which is well known to experts in the field continues to astound journalists and the general public.

Increased funding for social issues frequently follows heightened media attention. Between 1983 and 1989 in the United States, the amount of media coverage devoted to AIDS doubled every two years. Federal funds for AIDS research, education and testing increased at a similar rate, nearly doubling every two years.[21] As news coverage of TB in New York City quadrupled between 1984 and 1992, TB Cooperative Agreement appropriations for the city increased threefold over the same period.[22] When international media coverage on TB suddenly quadrupled from its level prior to 1992, the Global TB Programme budget also proceeded to quadruple over the next three years.[23] Certainly, many interrelated factors are involved in attracting donor support, though it is difficult to dispute that media coverage is often a major determinate.

Academic backlash

Scientific progress seems to be marked by one consistent law. The greater the utility of a discovery or breakthrough, the greater the skepticism and criticism it seems to trigger. Positive advances in the control of tuberculosis have not escaped this skepticism. When Robert Koch painstakingly presented the data of his discovery of the TB bacilli in Berlin, Germany's leading pathologist, Dr Rudolph Virchow, stormed out of the room in protest. Sir John Crofton's use of combination therapy to prevent drug resistance from developing and thereby increase the likelihood of cure was also dismissed by his peers.

So, there should be no surprise that a number of leading academics have greeted promotion of the DOTS strategy with vocal skepticism. Some critics have claimed that DOTS is a cumbersome, labor-intensive means of curing TB. They believe that it is impractical to observe every course of treatment for two months or longer. They argue that many countries lack the health infrastructure to provide such supervision.

This critique is largely based on the premise that society will continue to undervalue the lives of those suffering from TB, and that the political will to fund and expand the DOTS strategy will never be forthcoming. Indeed, the world's dismal track record of ignoring TB control argues for this analysis. Accordingly, some have concluded that the best hope for controlling TB lies in the development of a magic bullet in the form of a one-dose drug or effortless vaccine, even if the soonest possible date for discovering, testing and applying such a discovery is 15 to 20 years from now.

Hence, when WHO declared that the DOTS strategy represented 'the biggest health breakthrough of the 1990s' in terms of the number of lives it would be able to save, the reaction from a few leading researchers was swift and unqualified. Dr Barry Bloom of Albert Einstein College of Medicine dispatched an urgent appeal to the Programme to reverse its statement.

Dr Douglas Young of St. Mary's Hospital immediately resigned from a Global TB Programme advisory board in protest. According to Young, 'After decades of decline, there has been a renaissance in biomedical research on TB over the last five years. It would be very sad if promotion of DOTS was at the expense of neglecting this research effort.'[24]

Obviously, the solution is not to pit DOTS versus research into new and improved tools. The world must aggressively support both interventions. The DOTS strategy, if properly funded, can reduce TB deaths dramatically in the next decade. While this would represent an enormous accomplishment, better tools will ultimately be needed to eradicate tuberculosis from our planet. More than ever, funding for research is needed to more quickly extend the benefits of the DOTS strategy in the countries with the largest burden of TB cases. Better diagnostic techniques, quicker-acting medicines, innovative operational strategies and effective vaccines are needed to quickly draw the curtains on the TB epidemic before multidrug-resistant strains are given the opportunity to set the stage for an encore performance.

The future of political support for TB control

Unlike the political institutions waiting to take up the fight against tuberculosis, the bacilli themselves appear to be stubbornly apolitical in their mission. Nearly 30 million people are likely to die from tuberculosis in the next decade if DOTS is not used more widely. As many as 300 million additional people are likely to be infected with the TB bacilli during the same period of time. TB will continue to be the principal killer of HIV-positive people and will kill more women than all causes of maternal mortality combined. Especially hard-hit will be the emerging economies of Asia, which are increasingly becoming hot zones for MDR TB and global exporters of the virtually incurable disease.

But there are many hopeful signs that this particularly grim scenario can be avoided. The number of countries using WHO's recommended DOTS strategy has increased from 12 in 1993 to over 90 in 1998. More importantly, the number of TB patients annually receiving the DOTS strategy has increased nearly tenfold since a global TB emergency was declared, from approximately 100 000 patients before 1993 to around a million patients in 1998. However, this encouraging progress can obscure the more discouraging reality of how much more remains unaccomplished in the face of an enormous epidemic. As of 1998, only one in ten TB patients was covered by the DOTS strategy. The remaining nine in ten TB patients may still be receiving substandard treatment – or no treatment at all – and remain potential infectious threats to others. In spite of preliminary signs that TB control is becoming a higher political priority, this support can evaporate as quickly as it has appeared.

High-level political leadership is still being sought to spearhead the fight against TB. Efforts to use the DOTS strategy more widely are at a similar crossroads to that encountered in efforts to immunize children against diseases a decade ago. The turning point against childhood diseases was in 1984 when the Rockefeller Foundation sponsored the Bellagio conference and concrete plans were made by leading multilateral agencies to put existing, effective tools to wider use. As Bill Foege of the Carter Center recalls,

> When there is agreement of the experts, money will follow the plan. In 1984, Robert McNamara suggested that the agreements on immunization should lead us to seek $100 million in external funds each year for the global programme. Most people argued that such funds were unrealistic and if found would have to be taken from other health programmes. McNamara was correct and within three years no one would have settled any longer with $100 million per year.[25]

Within six years, immunization rates for children had increased from under 20 percent to nearly 80 percent.

A broader base of support from NGOs and other partners must also be mobilized to sustain efforts to use the DOTS strategy more widely and to reach the target of 70 percent DOTS coverage in the next decade. In an effort to catalyze this support, the first global World TB Day campaign was initiated on 24 March 1996, and has increasingly becoming a rallying point around the world for greater political commitment toward fighting TB. In the words of WHO's promotion materials, 'World TB Day is a time to demand that the effective tools and medicines discovered long ago be put to proper use.'[26] It is unlikely that health professionals alone will be able to make TB control a higher political priority unless support from a number of other sectors and ordinary citizens is also mobilized. As with child survival, it will take health and development generalists – more so than disease-specific specialists – to provide the political muscle to move control efforts forward.

The research community has a vital role in helping to ensure that the DOTS strategy is used more widely. Funding TB research at the US National Institutes for Health increased over eight-fold between 1991 and 1993, from $4.3 million to $35.9 million. Unfortunately, a disproportionate share of global TB research continues to mirror AIDS or cancer research strategies that presuppose that an effective cure does not already exist, rather than follow a leprosy or child survival research paradigm that investigates how to better utilize and improve existing, effective tools to quickly reduce morbidity and mortality. Certainly, basic research must be sustained, as the DOTS strategy can take the world a long way down the road to defeating tuberculosis, but not all of the way. To eventually eradicate TB, new drugs and vaccines will need to be developed. If this research is not begun immediately, there is little possibility that the world will have any additional tools at its disposal for widespread use by 2015. However, research institutions must also put their efforts behind expanding the DOTS strategy. As Reichman has observed, 'All the new tuberculosis drugs in the world will not cure tuberculosis in the 89 percent of patients lost to follow-up in the 1991 study in Harlem.'[27] The most pressing research needs are in the arena of operational research on the expansion of DOTS and community-based care, and in the development of quicker-acting diagnostic tools and fixed-dose combination therapies that are affordable for use in developing countries.

Ultimately, the governments of developing countries – particularly Ministries of Health and Ministries of Finance – and decision-makers in donor agencies control the future of the TB epidemic. They have the power to either send the TB epidemic dramatically into reverse, or permit it to worsen to the point where it is incurable and beyond control. Not surprisingly, many of the early pioneers who helped to develop the DOTS strategy have redirected their energies from solving therapeutic puzzles to discerning political agendas in these agencies. One such pioneer has been Sir John Crofton, who has taken the battle from the laboratory to the legislature. According to Crofton, 'Governments must be persuaded that they have a grim and urgent problem which is, nevertheless, soluble if quite modest national efforts and resources are devoted to it.'[28]

In conclusion, the reduction of tuberculosis cases in the next ten to twenty years is foremost a political challenge and a management challenge, more than a therapeutic or scientific challenge. Disproportionately, however, the resources, skills and strategies being applied to fight the epidemic are medical, and infrequently political or managerial. This can be seen at most national, regional or international TB conferences where discussion usually focuses on doctrinaire technical disputes over the efficacy of the BCG vaccine, tuberculin skin tests and chemoprophylaxis, and sorely neglects issues related to advocacy, social mobilization and human resource development. Moreover, the need for political support to fight tuberculosis must be sustained for decades. TB, the oldest recorded infectious disease, owes its longevity to its ability to remain dormant not only in the lungs, but also during society's fleeting, unsustained efforts at control and eradication.

Notes

1 According to the Centers for Disease Control, 'Three factors make this a realistic goal: 1) tuberculosis is retreating into geographically and demographically defined pockets; 2) biotechnology now has the potential for generating better diagnostic, treatment, and prevention modalities; and 3) computer, telecommunications, and other technologies can enhance technology transfer.' 'A Strategic Plan for the Elimination of Tuberculosis in the United States', in *Morbidity and Mortality Weekly Reports*, (21 April 1989), 38/S-3: 1.

2 *The News*, Islamabad, Pakistan, 11 April 1996.

3 Unforeseen by most. Exceptionally, Dr Georges Canetti anticipated the threat of the migration of populations and drug resistance in 1962, warning that 'there is no doubt that the principle factor preventing a decline in tuberculosis morbidity could one day be primary resistance'. Canetti then reaches a conclusion which is still lost on many health policy-makers over three decades later, 'On an international scale, among the efforts that are necessary to accomplish the eradication of tuberculosis, there is one absolute priority: the perfecting of chemotherapeutic methods adapted to conditions of "developing" countries. In realising this objective, the "developed" countries can give "developing" ones considerable help.' G. Canetti, 'The Eradication of Tuberculosis: Theoretical Problems and Practical Solutions', *Tubercle* 43 (1962) pp. 301–21.

4 The United States saw its TB death rate drop from around 200 annual deaths per 100 000 population in 1900 to around 50 in 1950. Because of the lack of surveillance data prior to 1900, it is difficult to assess what course the epidemic was taking in developing countries at the time. In some developing

countries, the epidemic may have been increasing. Puerto Rico, for example, saw annual death rates raise from approximately 150 in 1900 to around 250 a half century later. R. Dubos and J. Dubos, *The White Plague: Tuberculosis, Man, and Society* (Boston: Little, Brown, 1952).

5 *The Continuing Challenge of Tuberculosis* (Washington: Office of Technology Assessment, United States Congress, 1993).

6 J. P. Narain, M. C. Raviglione and A. Kochi, 'HIV-Associated Tuberculosis in Developing Countries: Epidemiology and Strategy for Prevention', *Tubercle and Lung Disease*, 73 (6) pp. 311–21; WHO country reports.

7 A. Mahmoudi and M. D. Iseman, 'Pitfalls in the Care of Patients with Tuberculosis', in *Journal of the American Medical Association* 270 (1993) pp. 65–8.

8 *Anti-Tuberculosis Drug Resistance in the World* (Geneva: World Health Organization, 1997).

9 From 1972 through 1982, TB control efforts were decentralized in the United States, and shifted to states in the form of block grants not earmarked for TB.

10 D. Bhatnagar, *Factors Influencing the Perceived Priority of Tuberculosis in India.* Unpublished project report submitted to the World Health Organization, 31 October 1996.

11 F. J. C. Millard, 'The Rising Incidence of Tuberculosis', in *Journal of the Royal Society of Medicine* (September, 1996) p. 89.

12 The ALA did continue to address the TB situation in the United States during this period of time, and has recently begun to become more involved in addressing the global TB situation.

13 Mario Raviglione, personal correspondence.

14 Dr Murdo Macdonald in a letter to the editor of the *Glasgow Herald*, 8 July 1997.

15 Christopher I. Holme, *Trial by TB: A Study in Current Attempts to Control the International Upsurge in Tuberculosis* (Edinburgh: Royal College of Physicians, 1997) p. 8.

16 IEC strategies educate and inform individuals about personal health choices and behavior, while advocacy strategies attempt to influence public policies and funding levels that affect the health of the community. IEC campaigns are usually targeted to the general public or to specific risk groups, while advocacy campaigns are usually targeted to encourage specific decision-makers to take action on a particular issue. Sometimes there is confusion between the two strategies as they both rely on media coverage, publications and coalition building, although with different audiences and intermediary objectives in mind.

17 Although this is beginning to change. One indication of this was the illness of New York Mets pitcher Jason Isringhauser who became sick with TB during the 1997 baseball season.

18 Thomas Frieden, correspondence, September 1996.

19 Ironically, the Global TB Programme has found that it has been able to *save* money by avoiding the preparation of exhaustive 200-page reports in favor of attractive, attention-getting 40-page reports which present messages in a way that they are more likely to be remembered.

20 Between 1989 and 1991, there were an average of 56 feature stories on tuberculosis annually in a group of a dozen leading international media outlets. Between 1992 and 1994, this increased to an average of 194 feature stories annually in the same group of media. The media surveyed include the *New*

York Times, Washington Post, Wall Street Journal, Los Angeles Times, Chicago Tribune, Associated Press, Inter Press Service, Reuters World Service, Manchester Guardian Weekly, The Economist, Time and *US News & World Report.*

21 E. Rogers, J. Dearing, and S. Chang, 'AIDS in the 1980s: the Agenda-Setting Process for a Public Issue', in *Journalism Monographs* 126 (April 1991) pp. 1–47.

22 Thomas Frieden, personal correspondence.

23 Global TB Programme annual reports; search of media coverage in leading international media outlets (see note 20) on Lexis-Nexis.

24 D. B. Young, 'New Tools for Tuberculosis Control: Do We Really Need Them?' in *The International Journal of Tuberculosis and Lung Disease* 1(3) (1997) p. 193.

25 W. H. Foege, 'Lessons From the Past', in J. D. H. Porter and K. P. W. J. MacAdam (eds), *Tuberculosis: Back to the Future* (Chichester: John Wiley, 1994).

26 WHO, *Guide to Obtaining Media Coverage* (1997).

27 L. B. Reichman, 'How to Ensure the Continued Resurgence of Tuberculosis', *The Lancet* (1996) 20 January, p. 347.

28 Sir John Crofton, 'Tuberculosis: World Perspective and the Challenges Ahead', *Journal of Pharmacy and Pharmacological Communications* 49, Suppl. 1, (1997) pp. 3–6.

6
Refugees and Migrants
Michael J. Toole

Introduction

The association between war and communicable diseases has been documented for many centuries. Combatants have been as likely to succumb to cholera, dysentery, or malaria as to the wounds of battle: for example, more than two-thirds of the estimated 660 000 deaths of soldiers in the American Civil War were caused by communicable diseases.[1] Moreover, the movements of military forces and the mass migrations of civilians due to war have often contributed to the spread of infectious agents into previously unexposed regions and populations. Since World War II, tens of millions of civilians have been forced to flee persecution or the violence of war to seek refuge either in neighbouring countries or in different areas of their own country. Most of these mass migrations have occurred in developing countries where the living conditions of the displaced have promoted the transmission of various communicable diseases. Since 1980, approximately 130 armed conflicts have occurred worldwide; 32 have each caused more than 1000 battlefield deaths.[2] In 1993 alone, 47 conflicts were active of which 43 were internal wars.[3] Armed conflicts have increasingly targeted civilian populations, resulting in high casualty rates, widespread human rights abuses, forced migration, and in some countries the total collapse of governance.

Refugees

Refugees who have crossed international borders fleeing war or persecution for reasons of race, religion, nationality, or membership in particular social and political groups are protected by several international conventions.[4] The number of refugees worldwide steadily increased from 5 million in 1980 to a peak of 21 million in August 1994 falling to approximately 16 million in 1996.[5] Since 1990 alone, more than 10 million refugees have been accorded protection and assistance by the international community. While most refugees are in Africa, the Middle East, and South Asia, there has been a rapid increase in the number of refugees in Europe since 1990. Almost two million refugees have been displaced within or have fled the republics of the former Yugoslavia.[6] Wars in the Azerbaijan enclave of Nagorno-Karabakh, ex-Soviet Georgia, and the rebellious Russian province of Chechnya have generated more than a million refugees.

Prior to 1990, most of the world's refugees fled countries that ranked among the poorest in the world, such as Afghanistan, Cambodia, Mozambique and Ethiopia. However, during this decade, an increasing number of refugees have originated in relatively more affluent countries, such as Kuwait, Iraq, the former Yugoslavia, and Armenia. Nevertheless, the reasons for the flight of refugees generally remain the same: war, civil strife and persecution. Hunger, while sometimes a primary cause of population movements, is all too frequently only a contributing factor. For example, during 1992, although severe drought in southern Africa and the Horn of Africa affected food production in all countries in those regions, only in war-torn Mozambique and Somalia did millions of hungry inhabitants migrate in search of food.

While many people fled the generalized violence of war, most fled because they were specifically targeted by one or another armed faction. Civilians in Somalia have been targeted by armed militia because of their membership in a patrilineal clan; Muslim Rohingyas of Burma were victims of religious persecution by their government; ethnic Nepalis were harassed by Bhutanese authorities; Liberians were attacked or murdered because of their ethnicity; and Croatians, Serbs, and Bosnian Muslims were victims of ancient ethnic and religious feuds.

The most dramatic example of a mass refugee exodus occurred in 1994 following the attempted genocide of the Tutsi minority by extremist elements of the Hutu majority in Rwanda. Initially, more than 500 000 refugees fled into Burundi and Tanzania; later, in July, when the Rwandan Patriotic Front militarily defeated the Rwandan government and took over the country, one million ethnic Hutus abruptly fled to eastern Zaire provoking an unprecedented refugee crisis. In late 1996, this mass migration was repeated in the reverse direction when most of the refugees abruptly returned to their homeland following, on one side of the country, armed conflict in eastern Zaire between rebels and Zairean Government forces, and on the other, insistence by the Tanzanian Government that the refugees return home.

Internally displaced persons

In addition to those persons who meet the international definition of refugees, an estimated 25 million people have fled their homes for the same reasons as refugees but remain internally displaced in their countries of origin.[7] Most internally displaced persons are found in sub-Saharan Africa, the Middle East, the former Yugoslavia, and the republics of the former Soviet Union. Internally displaced persons are often more vulnerable to both human rights abuses and adverse health consequences because they are not provided the same degree of international protection as refugees and access to them by humanitarian relief agencies is often difficult and dangerous.

Risk factors

A new term – *complex emergency* – has been coined to describe situations affecting large civilian populations which usually involve a combination of factors including war or civil strife, food shortages and population displacement, resulting in significant excess mortality.

The conditions that lead to widespread outbreaks of communicable diseases among refugees and internally displaced persons develop gradually as the situation in their country deteriorates. Political instability, the persecution of certain minorities, and human rights abuses lead to civil unrest and violence. Governments and ruling elites respond with greater repression, causing widespread armed conflict. The direct destruction of infrastructure, the diversion of resources away from community services, and general economic collapse lead to a deterioration in medical services, especially prevention programmes such as child immunization and antenatal care. Medical treatment facilities are overwhelmed by the needs of war casualties; the routine management of medical problems suffers from lack of staff and shortages in essential medical supplies. For example, the major hospital in the central Bosnian city of Zenica reported that the proportion of all surgical cases associated with trauma steadily increased from 22 per cent in April 1992, at the beginning of the war, reaching 78 per cent in November of the same year.[8]

Deliberate diversion of food supplies by various armed factions, disruption of transport and marketing, and economic hardship often cause severe food deficits. Local farmers may not plant crops as extensively as usual, the supply of seeds and fertilizer may be disrupted, irrigation systems may be damaged by the fighting, and crops may be intentionally destroyed or looted by armed soldiers. In countries that do not normally produce agricultural surpluses or that have large pastoral or nomadic communities, the impact of food deficits on the nutritional status of civilians may be severe, particularly in sub-Saharan Africa. If adverse climatic factors intervene, as often happens in drought-prone countries such as Sudan, Somalia, Mozambique and Ethiopia, the outcome may be catastrophic. High rates of acute malnutrition have been documented among children less than five years of age in many refugee and internally displaced populations.[9] The relationship between malnutrition and infection is well known; communicable disease case fatality rates are higher among malnourished children than among the well-nourished, and diseases such as acute diarrhoea and measles may contribute to the malnourished state.

In some countries, such as Liberia and Somalia, governance has completely collapsed and the normal functions of a modern nation-state have ceased. Most public services, including health and education, cease to be delivered on a national scale. When this degree of anarchy develops, the provision of effective humanitarian assistance becomes logistically difficult and extremely dangerous for relief personnel. Relief convoys are prey to bandits and local warlords, massive diversion of relief supplies occurs, and the implementation of sustainable, community-supported programmes becomes virtually impossible. The proliferation and loose control of weapons in many countries have compounded the problem. In many developing nations, growth in military spending has far exceeded domestic economic growth rates. One study found that 29 of 134 surveyed countries spent a greater proportion of their national budget on the military than on health and education combined.[10]

Public health impact

Mass movements of refugees and internally displaced persons have had severe public health consequences. These populations have often been located in remote, crowded and unhygienic camps with inadequate food, clean water, and sanitation facilities. A high proportion of refugees and displaced persons in developing countries have been children; moreover, the high prevalence of acute protein-energy malnutrition among young children has increased their vulnerability to adverse outcomes from infectious diseases.

Mortality

The most reliable estimates of mortality rates have come from well-defined and secure refugee camps where there is a reasonable level of camp organization and a designated agency has had responsibility for the collection of data. The most difficult situations have been those where internally displaced persons have been scattered over a wide area and where surveys could take place only in relatively secure zones. Mortality rates have been estimated from hospital and burial records, community-based surveys, and 24-hour burial site surveillance. Early in an emergency, when mortality rates are elevated, it is useful to express the crude mortality rate (CMR) as deaths per 10 000 population per day. In most developing countries, the baseline annual CMR in non-refugee populations has been reported between 12 and 20 per 1000, corresponding to a daily rate of approximately 0.3–0.6 per 10 000. A threshold of one per 10 000 per day has been used commonly to define an elevated CMR and to characterize a situation as an emergency.[11]

During the past 20 years, crude mortality rates as high as 30 times baseline rates have not been unusual during the first month or two following an acute movement of refugees.

Refugees are usually at highest risk of mortality during the period immediately after their arrival in the country of asylum, reflecting long periods of inadequate food and medical care prior to, or during, their flight. For example, during July and August 1992, the daily CMR among Mozambican refugees who had been in the Zimbabwean camp of Chambuta for less than one month was 8 per 10 000 population. This was four times the death rate of refugees who had been in the camp between one and three months, and 16 times the death rate normally reported for non-displaced populations in Mozambique.[12]

Following the massive influx of Rwandan refugees into the North Kivu region of eastern Zaire in July 1994, the daily CMR based on body counts ranged between 25 and 50 per 10 000 per day. The difficulty in estimating the size of the refugee population (the denominator for rate calculations) accounted for the wide range of estimates. Population surveys conducted in the refugee camps, which provided mortality estimates independent of population size, found that between 7 per cent and 9 per cent of the refugees died during the first month after the influx.

Communicable diseases

The most common causes of morbidity and mortality among refugees during the early influx phase have been diarrhoeal diseases, measles, acute respiratory infections, malaria, and other infectious diseases.[13] These diseases – as well as acute malnutrition – have been the focus of most public health interventions. In some settings, most deaths could be attributed to one or two communicable diseases. In the Goma camps of eastern Zaire, for example, more than 90 per cent of the estimated

50 000 deaths in the first month after the refugee influx were caused by either watery or bloody diarrhoea.[14] During 1992–3, when attention was focused on the provision of food to war-affected populations in Somalia, between 53 per cent and 81 per cent of deaths documented in population surveys were attributed to either measles or diarrhoeal disease.

Diarrhoeal diseases

Diarrhoeal diseases have consistently been among the top two or three causes of mortality in refugee and displaced populations in developing countries. While most deaths have probably not been caused by cholera or Shiga dysentery, the spread of these two diseases has been promoted by mass forced migrations, especially in Africa and the Middle East. Of considerable concern is the rapid development of multiple antibiotic resistance by *Shigella dysenteriae* type I in Central Africa, a process that has accelerated during the conflicts and migrations of the past five years.

The political nature of cholera was illustrated in 1985 by an outbreak which occurred among Ethiopian military forces who were engaged in civil conflicts on several fronts. The Ethiopian government at the time did not report the outbreak and denied that cholera was present in the country. Consequently, control efforts were ineffective and the epidemic spread rapidly to refugee populations in neighboring Somalia and eastern Sudan.[15]

When approximately 400 000 Kurdish refugees fled Iraqi cities in 1991 and found refuge in squalid camps on the Turkish border, more than 70 per cent of deaths were associated with diarrhoea, including cholera.[16] Cholera epidemics have occurred in refugee camps in Malawi, Zimbabwe, Swaziland, Somalia, Sudan, Nepal, Bangladesh, Turkey, Afghanistan, Burundi and Zaire.[17] An extensive epidemic affected most of the war-affected southern regions of Somalia in 1993 and 1994. Studies have identified risk factors for cholera infection in refugee camps that include: drinking water from rivers or shallow wells, lacking water containers of adequate size, inadequately protected water storage containers, and having insufficient cooking pots.[18] Cholera case–fatality rates in refugee camps have ranged between 3 per cent and 30 per cent, depending on the degree of preparedness.

In the Goma area of eastern Zaire, an explosive cholera outbreak occurred within the first week of the arrival of refugees in July 1994. This outbreak was associated with rapid faecal contamination of the alkaline water of Lake Kivu which was the primary source of drinking water for the refugees. The organism responsible for the epidemic was resistant to commonly used antibiotics such as tetracycline and doxy-cycline. Facility-based CFRs were as high as 22 per cent during the early days of the epidemic; however, once adequate relief personnel arrived and treatment resources were obtained, the CFR dropped rapidly to 2–3 per cent.[19] As the cholera outbreak subsided, an equally lethal epidemic of dysentery occurred. Consequently, over 90 per cent of deaths in the first month after the influx were attributed to diarrhoeal disease. When hundreds of thousands of Rwandans returned to their country in late 1996, only sporadic cases of cholera were reported.

In eastern Europe, cholera outbreaks in Armenia, Azerbaijan, Georgia, the Central Asian Republics, and the southern regions of the Russian Federation have been associated with civil conflict and the movement of refugees between the states of the former Soviet Union and in and out of Afghanistan. In the former Yugoslavia, cholera was not reported during the war. However, after the war began in Bosnia and Herzegovina in 1992, the quantity and quality of urban water supplies deteriorated as a result of diverted water sources, cracked water pipes, lack of diesel fuel to run water pumps, and frequent losses of water pressure that, in turn, caused cross-contamination by sewage. In August 1993, piped water supplies in the capital Sarajevo were restricted to an average of 5 litres per person per day (the Office of the United Nations High Commis-sioner for Refugees [UNHCR] recommends daily minimum provision of at least 15 litres per person). Consequently, in Sarajevo between January and June 1993, the incidence of diarrhoea and dysentery increased sevenfold and twelvefold, respectively.[20]

Since 1991, explosive outbreaks of dysentery caused by *Shigella dysenteriae* type I have been reported among refugees and internally displaced persons in Malawi, Nepal, Kenya, Bangladesh, Burundi, Rwanda, Tanzania and Zaire.[21] Dysentery attack rates have been as high as 32 per cent and case–fatality rates have been as high as 10 per cent in young children and the elderly.[22] Resistance to cotrimoxasole and nalidixic acid was reported in Rwanda, Burundi, and Zaire and rates of compliance to the five-day regimen of ciprofloxacin were reported to be low in Rwandan camps for refugees from Burundi.[23] The effective prevention and treatment of *Shigella dysenteriae* type I has emerged as one of the leading public health challenges among refugee and displaced populations in Central Africa.

Measles

Outbreaks of measles within refugee camps were common prior to 1990 and caused many deaths. Low levels of immunization coverage, coupled with high rates of undernutrition and vitamin A deficiency, played a critical role in the spread of measles and the subsequent mortality within some refugee camps. Measles has been one of the leading causes of death among children in refugee camps; in addition, measles has contributed to high malnutrition rates among those who have survived the initial illness. Measles infection may lead to or exacerbate vitamin A deficiency, compromising immunity and leaving the patient susceptible to xerophthalmia, blindness, and premature death. In early 1985, the measles-specific death rate among children under 5 in one eastern Sudan camp was 30 per 1000 per month; the CFR based on reported cases was almost 30 per cent.[24] Large numbers of measles deaths have been reported in camps in Somalia, Bangladesh, Sudan and Ethiopia.[25] Since 1990, mass immunization campaigns have been effective in reducing the measles morbidity and mortality rates in refugee camps: for example, in Zaire, Tanzania, Burundi and Malawi. Measles outbreaks probably did not occur during other major refugee emergencies (e.g. Somalis in Ethiopia in 1989; Iraqis in Turkey in 1991) because immunization coverage rates were already high in those refugee populations prior to their flight.[26]

Malaria

Mass migration and malaria have been closely associated in recent decades. Some of the major epidemics of malaria and the most severe forms of drug resistance have occurred in border regions with high numbers of refugees, such as the borders between Thailand and Burma, Thailand and Cambodia, and Ethiopia and Sudan. Malaria has caused high rates of morbidity and mortality among refugees and displaced persons in countries where malaria is endemic, such as Thailand, eastern Sudan, Somalia, Kenya, Malawi, Zimbabwe, Burundi, Rwanda and Zaire.[27] Malaria-specific mortality rates have been especially high when refugees from areas of low malaria endemicity have fled through, or into, areas of high endemicity. Recent examples include the movement of Cambodian refugees through highly endemic areas into Thailand in 1979, the influx of highland Ethiopians into eastern Sudan in 1985, and the exodus of highland Rwandans into Zaire in 1994. The severity of malaria outbreaks in Africa has been exacerbated by the rapid spread of chloroquine resistance during the 1980s. In eastern Sudan, for example, the development of chloroquine resistance coincided with the expansion of camps for Eritrean refugees many of whom had not previously been exposed to malaria resulting in explosive outbreaks of severe disease during the late 1980s. Cross-border movements of refugees probably contributed to the introduction of chloroquine-resistant malaria into Eritrea. In addition, resistance to sulfadoxine-pyrimethamine has also been reported among Rwandan refugees in eastern Zaire since 1994 and resistance to mefloquine has been documented among Burmese refugees in Thailand.[28]

Malaria has been extensively documented as a major health problem among military forces serving in foreign wars, including Allied personnel in World Wars I and II, Americans in the Korean and Vietnam Wars, and Soviet forces in Afghanistan.[29] However, there is no evidence that imported malaria cases among either military personnel or refugees has led to indigenous transmission in countries where malaria has been eradicated.

Meningitis

A different form of migration has been associated with the rapid spread of a new epidemic and invasive form of *Neisseria meningitidis*, Group A. The strain (A:4:P1.9/clone III- 1) was first isolated during a meningitis outbreak in 1987 at the annual Islamic pilgrimage in Makkah, Saudi Arabia. This strain is responsible for the second meningococcal pandemic in Africa and has been associated with epidemics in Cameroon, Chad, Niger, Togo, Central African Republic, Burkino Faso, and other countries.[30]

The crowding associated with refugee camps places refugees at high risk of meningococcal meningitis in endemic areas, particularly in countries within or near the traditionally described 'meningitis belt' of sub-Saharan Africa.[31] Outbreaks have been reported in Malawi, Ethiopia, Burundi and Zaire; however, mass immunization has proved to be an effective epidemic control measure in these situations and meningococcal morbidity and mortality rates have been relatively low. In the Zairean camp of Kibumba, the incidence reached 19 per 100 000 during the week of 8–14 August 1994, resulting in a mass vaccination campaign which successfully averted a wider epidemic.[32]

Hepatitis E

The spread of enterically-transmitted hepatitis non-A, non-B in east Africa has been largely the result of mass migrations due to wars in the region. Refugees in camps in Somalia (1986), Ethiopia (1989), and Kenya (1991) have experienced outbreaks with attack rates between 6 per cent and 8 per cent, and case–fatality rates among pregnant women between 14 per cent and 17 per cent.[33] The Kenya outbreak was the first in which infection with the hepatitis E virus was confirmed: between

March and October 1991, one in five deaths in the Somali refugee camp of Liboi in Kenya were attributed to this disease.[34] The political instability, armed conflict and population migrations that marked Somalia in the late 1980s and early 1990s were associated with numerous hepatitis E epidemics. One such outbreak was reported in villages along the Shebeli River in the Lower Shebeli region in 1988–9. A total of 11 413 cases of icteric hepatitis were identified (an attack rate of 4.6 per cent), with 346 deaths (a case–fatality rate of 3.0 per cent). Anti-HEV was found in 128 of 145 (88 per cent) people sampled. The case–fatality rate in pregnant females was 13.8 per cent.[35]

Tuberculosis

In complex emergencies when basic health services have been disrupted, treatment of patients with active tuberculosis may be inadequate or incomplete, leading potentially to increased transmission in affected communities. During the war years in Bosnia and Herzegovina between 1992 and 1995, the incidence of new cases of tuberculosis reportedly increased fourfold.[36] Likewise, in Somalia during the civil war and famine of 1991–2, routine case-finding, treatment and follow-up of tuberculosis patients almost ceased. Consequently, there was a marked increase in both the incidence of new cases and the tuberculosis-related CFR.[37] A study in El Salvador showed that the incidence of smear-positive pulmonary tuberculosis among persons displaced by the war in the 1980s was three times the rate in the non-displaced. The annual risk of tuberculosis infection showed a steady increase during the latter six years of the war reaching a high 2.3 per cent in 1992.[38]

Tuberculosis is well recognized as a health problem among refugee and displaced populations. The crowded living conditions and underlying poor nutritional status of refugee populations may foster the spread of the disease. Although not a leading cause of mortality during the emergency phase, tuberculosis often emerges as a critical problem once measles and diarrhoeal diseases have been adequately controlled. For example, in 1985, 26 per cent and 38 per cent, respectively, of adult deaths among refugees in Somalia and eastern Sudan were attributed to tuberculosis.[39] The high prevalence of HIV infection among many African refugee populations may contribute to the high rate of transmission.

Tuberculosis among migrants and refugees who have been resettled in western industrialized countries has received a lot of attention and is described in a large body of published literature. In countries such as the United States, Canada, Australia, France, and the Scandinavian states, a large proportion of new cases of tuberculosis occurs among recently arrived immigrants and refugees. For example, in the Australian state of Victoria, 80 per cent of newly notified cases in 1990 were among persons born overseas compared with only 40 per cent in 1970.[40] Between 1987 and 1991, the mean annual incidence of tuberculosis in Victorian residents born in Australia and Southeast Asia was 1.5 and 47.5 per 100 000 respectively. The incidence of multi-drug resistance was reported to have remained at a steady 2 per cent during the past 15 years and appears not to have been influenced by the influx of refugees and immigrants from high prevalence countries.

HIV infection and other sexually transmitted diseases

HIV infection and other STDs may be a problem associated with complex emergencies, especially when there is a breakdown in routine medical services. Several recent mass population migrations have taken place in areas where HIV infection prevalence rates are high, for example, in Burundi, Rwanda, Malawi, Ethiopia and Zaire. One study provided convincing data to suggest that the geographical spread of HIV infection in Uganda correlated with the ethnic patterns of recruitment into the Ugandan National Liberation Army in the late 1970s.[41] In one of the few refugee populations studied for this infection, the HIV prevalence among adult male Sudanese refugees in western Ethiopia was 7 per cent; the prevalence of infection among commercial sex workers living in the vicinity of the camp was greater than 40 per cent.[42] Serological surveys in this population also revealed high rates of previous infection with syphilis and chancroid. The contribution of HIV infection to morbidity and mortality among refugees has not been documented, but may be significant. In the former Yugoslavia, there have been many reports of sexual assault and increased prostitution; in addition, high rates of violence-related trauma have increased the rate of blood transfusions.[43] In this setting, where shortages of laboratory reagents to test blood for HIV are widespread, the risk of increased transmission of HIV is high, though this trend has not yet been confirmed by studies.

Other infectious diseases

A massive epidemic of visceral leishmaniasis (*kala-azar*) occurred between 1989 and 1992 among populations affected by the civil war in southern Sudan. Treatment was available only in limited areas and the disease spread to Western Upper Nile province which was not known previously to be endemic for *kala-azar*.[44] More than one million southern Sudanese migrated to the northern part of the country and more than 600 were treated for *kala-azar* in Khartoum between January 1989 and February

1990.[45] Sudanese refugees transmitted the disease to camps in the Gambela Region of Western Ethiopia.[46] Rickettsial infections have been among the most feared communicable diseases in refugee and war-affected populations. However, few reports have documented outbreaks during the past 20 years. Murine and scrub typhus were reported among Cambodian refugees in camps on the Thai-Cambodian border[47] and an epidemic of louse-borne typhus was reported in four provinces of war-torn Burundi in early 1997 (unpublished data, World Health Organization, February 1997).

Discussion

War, famine and mass forced migrations have been associated throughout history with epidemics of infectious diseases. In recent decades, the impact of outbreaks of infectious diseases has been documented in many populations of refugees and internally displaced persons. Much of the excess mortality related to mass migration has been attributed to diarrhoeal diseases, measles, malaria, meningitis, and other infectious diseases. Even among non-displaced communities in war zones, the incidence of infectious diseases has increased due to the collapse of basic preventive and clinical services. These trends have been most marked in developing countries where living conditions and limited social services have increased the risk of transmission and the severity of clinical outcomes.

The contribution of migration to the spread of infectious diseases beyond the directly affected populations has been less well documented. It seems likely that the movement of refugees and internally displaced persons has contributed to the spread of multi-drug resistant epidemic bacillary dysentery in Central Africa; the rapid transmission of hepatitis E virus infection in East Africa; and cholera in Africa and the former Soviet Union. The increased incidence of severe malaria in certain border regions has largely been due to the movement of non-immune populations *into* areas of high endemicity. There is little evidence that refugees have introduced the malaria parasite or increased the level of transmission of malaria within the local population of the country where they have sought asylum. However, refugees returning to their countries of origin may have helped introduce drug-resistant malaria in their home communities. The rapid spread of visceral leishmaniasis in Sudan and to a lesser extent in western Ethiopia during the 1980s and early 1990s was associated with the civil conflict in southern Sudan and the subsequent collapse of medical services and mass population displacement.

The peaceful movement of large numbers of Islamic pilgrims to and from the Saudi holy city of Makkah undoubtedly contributed to the spread of a new strain of meningococcal meningitis which is now held responsible for a second pandemic of the disease in and beyond sub-Saharan Africa's so-called meningitis belt. The rapid global spread of the human immunodeficiency virus since the late 1970s has been due to travel by large numbers of individuals for a range of commercial and tourist purposes rather than to mass forced migrations of the kind discussed above. Although there is some evidence that military forces have contributed to the spread of HIV, there is no evidence that refugees have significantly contributed to increased transmission of the virus in the countries where they have sought refuge. On the contrary, refugees may be at heightened risk of infection if they are exposed to the following risk factors: health services where universal precautions against infection are not practised; sexual exploitation or rape; and/or lack of preventive education and condoms.

Likewise, although the incidence of newly diagnosed tuberculosis is relatively high among recent immigrants in industrialized countries, there is no evidence that this has led to increased transmission among native-born residents. Moreover, the incidence of new cases of TB among Southeast and South Asian immigrants in these settings is significantly lower than the rate in their countries of origin. Overall recent increases in TB incidence and the development of multiple drug resistance reported in some countries, such as the United States, is related more to social constraints to case-finding and treatment compliance and to the AIDS epidemic than to immigration from countries of high TB prevalence.

There are two key issues for discussion. Firstly, mortality rates among refugees and internally displaced persons are often unacceptably high, especially in developing countries, and most of this mortality has been due to preventable communicable diseases. Secondly, armed conflict and mass forced migration has been associated with the spread of certain communicable diseases, in particular multiple drug-resistant forms of these diseases. Addressing the first issue will probably deal effectively with the second. The prevention of excess mortality among refugee and displaced populations requires three strategies which could be characterized in a medical model as primary, secondary and tertiary prevention. Primary prevention involves conflict resolution and the protection of civilian populations affected by war. Secondary prevention consists of emergency preparedness and the provision of adequate food, water, shelter and sanitation to refugees and internally displaced persons.

Tertiary prevention comprises medical measures to prevent and manage those communicable diseases that have been identified as the key threats.

Primary prevention

The most urgent need is to develop more effective diplomatic and political mechanisms that might resolve conflicts early in their evolution prior to the stage when food shortages occur, health services collapse, populations migrate, and significant adverse public health outcomes emerge. One of the major obstacles is the almost sacred notion of national sovereignty embodied in the United Nations Charter. The prohibition against the threat or use of force on the territory of independent sovereign member-states of the United Nations has forced the international community to stand by and watch extreme examples of human rights abuses until, in certain cases, a threshold of tolerance has been crossed and public indignation has demanded action, as in the case of Somalia. By the time such action has been taken, the conflict has often advanced to a stage where any involvement by outside forces is perceived by belligerents as taking sides, thereby entangling the international community in the conflict itself, as occurred in Somalia. Cautious, neutral, but determined diplomacy of the kind practiced by the Atlanta-based Carter Center in Ethiopia, Sudan, Haiti, and Bosnia-Herzegovina might serve as a model for future conflict resolution efforts. Epidemiologists and behavioural scientists might play a role in this process by systematically studying the dynamics and characteristic behaviours that sustain conflict situations and by seeking to identify measures that might reduce the level of tension between opposing sides.

Secondary prevention

Preparedness planning for complex emergencies needs to take place both at a coordinated international level and at the individual country level. The international community would be wise to invest funds in strengthening the existing network of experienced relief organizations. These agencies need resources to implement early warning systems, maintain technical expertise, train personnel, build reserves of relief supplies, and develop their logistic capacity. At the country level, all health development programmes should have an emergency preparedness component which should include the establishment of standard public health policies (for example, immunization and management of epidemics), treatment protocols, staff training, and the maintenance of reserves of essential drugs and vaccines for use in disasters.

Early warning systems need to be strengthened. Emergency detection activities in the form of early warning systems and risk-mapping have existed for some time; however, these systems have tended to focus on monitoring natural rather than manmade hazards. These systems have not developed early indicators related to human rights abuses, ethnic conflict, political instability, and migration. Groups such as Africa Watch, Physicians for Human Rights, Amnesty International, and African Rights have conducted assessments of vulnerability in countries, such as Burundi, relatively early in the evolution of civil conflict. The problem with such assessments is that the results are often ignored by the governments of wealthy donor nations if perceived not to be in their security interests. Epidemiologists, economists, agronomists, and other specialists may play an important role in developing and field testing the sensitivity and specificity of a broad range of early warning indicators that are better predictors than the late indicators, such as mortality rates and malnutrition prevalence, that are traditionally measured by population surveys.

In the absence of conflict resolution, those communities that are totally dependent on external aid for their survival, because they have either been displaced from their homes or are living under a state of siege, must be provided the basic minimum resources necessary to maintain health and well-being. The provision of adequate food, clean water, shelter, sanitation and warmth will prevent the most severe public health consequences of complex emergencies. Minimum standards for the quantity and quality of food rations and water in emergency settings have long been established.[48]

Tertiary prevention

Appropriate interventions for the prevention of specific communicable diseases must be implemented promptly. Immunization of children against measles is probably the single most important (and cost-effective) preventive measure in emergency-affected populations, particularly those housed in camps. Immunization programmes should eventually include all antigens recommended by WHO's Expanded Programme on Immunization. The traditional parenteral cholera vaccine often used in epidemic settings in the past was only 50 per cent effective in preventing cholera and is no longer recommended by WHO.[49] Of the two newer and potentially effective vaccines currently available, one requires two doses and does not induce immunity until 7–10 days after the second dose; the other, a single-dose, oral, live vaccine, has never been subjected to testing under field conditions and its use in emergency-affected populations would be controversial. Thus, mass vaccination is currently not considered to be an effective cholera epidemic control measure in these settings. A public health surveillance system is an essential part of the relief program and should be established immediately.[50] Malaria control in refugee camps is difficult. Under the transient circumstances that characterize most refugee camps, vector control techniques have generally been impractical and expensive. Prompt identification and treatment of symptomatic individuals is a more effective measure to reduce malaria mortality, although the spread of chloroquine resistance means that effective case management will become more expensive and technically more challenging in the future.

Appropriate curative programmes with adequate population coverage need to be instituted. An essential drug list and standardized treatment protocols are necessary elements of a curative programme. It is not necessary to develop totally new guidelines in each refugee situation: several excellent manuals already exist, from which guidelines can be adapted to suit local conditions.[51] WHO has also developed guidelines for the clinical management of dehydration from diarrhoea and for acute respiratory infections that can be used by trained community health workers (CHWs).[52] Some relief programmes, such as those in Somalia, Sudan, and Malawi have successfully trained large numbers of refugees as CHWs to detect cases of diarrhoea and ARI, provide primary treatment, and refer severely ill patients to a clinic, thereby increasing coverage by health services and diminishing reliance on expatriate workers.

The front-line relief workers in complex emergencies are often volunteers recruited by non-governmental organizations (NGOs) who sometimes lack specific training and experience in emergency relief. They require knowledge and practical experience in a broad range of subjects, including food and nutrition, water and sanitation, disease surveillance, immunization, communicable disease control, epidemic management, and maternal and child health care. They should be able to conduct rapid public health needs assessments, establish priorities, work closely with affected communities, train local workers, coordinate with a complex array of relief organizations, monitor and evaluate the impact of their activities, and efficiently manage scarce resources. In addition, they need to function effectively in an often hostile and dangerous environment; such skills are specific to emergencies and are not necessarily present in the average graduate of a Western medical or nursing school. Therefore, relief agencies need to allocate more resources to relevant training and orientation of their staff, as well as providing adequate support in the field.

Since the end of the Cold War, the military forces of various nations have played an increasingly visible role in providing emergency humanitarian assistance. The involvement of the military is often ambiguous, confusing the various tasks of peace-keeping, peace-enforcing, and providing relief. No one would doubt the logistical advantages of the military; however, this is not always matched with appropriate experience in the technical aspects of a relief operation. Furthermore, military assistance is expensive; for example, in the Rwandan camps of eastern Zaire each US soldier involved in providing clean water to the refugees was accompanied by a squad of armed soldiers for his protection. Finally, because military deployment depends on political decisions by national governments, it cannot always be integrated into disaster preparedness planning.

Although existing technical knowledge is sufficient to prevent much of the morbidity and mortality associated with mass displacement, refugees and internally displaced persons will continue to find refuge in remote regions where the provision of basic needs requires creative approaches. Therefore, there is a need for systematic operational and evaluation research in certain areas of nutrition (for example, effective methods of preventing micronutrient deficiency diseases), water supply and disease control. Greater resources need to be allocated to personnel training, emergency preparedness planning and the maintenance of regional reserves of essential relief supplies. These activities need to include government and non-government agencies in developing countries where emergencies are likely to occur. The increasingly favoured option of military intervention often reflects the lack of attention given to conflicts in the early stages of their evolution. Determined diplomacy applied early in a conflict might preclude the need for later military toughness, with all the associated problems observed recently in Somalia.

Finally, we must be careful that the link between mass migration and epidemics of communicable diseases is not used to impede the free movement of populations that genuinely seek refuge from persecution and violence. Refugees are not the problem; the real problem lies in the unchecked spread of violence that leads to their migration and the lack of consistency in the approach by the international community to the resolution of conflict and the protection of innocent civilian populations. By developing sensitive and accurate early warning systems, carefully documenting the public health consequences of emergencies, and designing effective, focused assistance programmes, public health professionals may act as credible advocates for prompt humanitarian responses at the highest levels of political decision-making. The impact of mass migration on the spread of epidemic communicable diseases can be minimized by addressing the root causes of civil conflict, ensuring adequate protection of civilian populations, and implementing proven preventive programmes for refugees and internally displaced persons.

Notes

1 J. S. Sartin, 'Infectious Diseases During the Civil War: the Triumph of the Third Army', *Clinical Infectious Diseases*, 16 (1993) pp. 580–4.

2 J. Cobey, A. Flanigin and W. Foege, 'Effective Humanitarian Aid: Our Only Hope for Intervention in Civil War', *Journal of the American Medical Association* (hereafter *JAMA*), 270 (1993) pp. 632–4.

3 P. Wallenstein and K. Axell, 'Conflict Resolution and the End of the Cold War, 1989–93', *Journal of Peace Research*, 31 (1994) pp. 333–49.

4 United Nations High Commissioner for Refugees, *Convention and Protocol Relating to the Status of Refugees*, HCR/INF/29/Rev 3 (Geneva: WHO, 1992).

5 US Committee for Refugees, *World Refugee Survey, 1996* (Washington, DC).

6 US Committee for Refugees, *World Refugee Survey, 1995* (Washington, DC).

7 *World Refugee Survey 1996*, op. cit.

8 Centers for Disease Control and Prevention, 'Status of Public Health, Bosnia and Herzegovina, August–September 1993', *Mortality and Morbidity Weekly Report* (hereafter *MMWR*), 973 (1993) pp. 979–82.

9 Centers for Disease Control and Prevention, 'Famine-Affected, Refugee and Displaced Populations: Recommendations for Public Health Issues', *MMWR*, 41 (1993) RR-13.

10 A. Zwi and A. Ugalde, 'Political Violence in the Third World: a Public Health Issue', *Health Policy and Planning*, 6 (1991) pp. 203–17.

11 'Famine-Affected, Refugee and Displaced Populations', op. cit.

12 Centers for Disease Control and Prevention, 'Mortality among Newly-Arrived Mozambican Refugees, Zimbabwe and Malawi, 1992', *MMWR*, 42 (1993) pp. 468–9; 475–7.

13 'Famine-Affected, Refugee and Displaced Populations', op. cit.

14 Goma Epidemiology Group, 'Public Health Impact of Rwandan Refugee Crisis: What Happened in Goma, Zaire, in July 1994?' *Lancet*, 345 (1995) pp. 339–44.

15 K. Mulholland, 'Cholera in Sudan: an Account of an Epidemic in a Refugee Camp in Eastern Sudan, May–June 1985', *Disasters*, 9 (1985) pp. 247–58.

16 Centers for Disease Control and Prevention, 'Public Health Consequences of Acute Displacement of Iraqi Citizens: March–May 1991', *MMWR*, 40 (1991) pp. 443–6.

17 'Famine-Affected, Refugee and Displaced Populations', op. cit.; 'Public Health Impact of Rwandan Refugee Crisis', op. cit.

18 A. Moren, S. Stefanaggi, D. Antona, D. Bitar, M. G. Etchegorry, M. Tchatchioka, G. Lungu, 'Practical Field Epidemiology to Investigate a Cholera Outbreak in a Mozambican Refugee Camp in Malawi, 1988', *Journal of Tropical Medicine and Hygiene*, 94 (1991) pp. 1–7; D. L. Hatch, R. J. Waldman, G. W. Lungu, C. Piri, 'Epidemic Cholera during Refugee Resettlement in Malawi', *International Journal of Epidemiology*, 23 (1994) pp. 1292–9.

19 'Public Health Impact of Rwanden Refugee Crisis', op. cit.

20 'Status of Public Health, Bosnia and Herzegovina', op. cit.

21 'Famine-Affected, Refugee and Displaced Populations', op. cit.; 'Public Health Impact of Rwandan Refugee Crisis', op. cit.; Centers for Disease Control and Prevention, 'Health Status of Displaced Persons Following Civil War: Burundi, December 1993 – January 1994', *MMWR*, 43 (1994) pp. 701–1.

22 'Burundi, December 1993', ibid.

23 J. D. Cavallo, L. Niel, A. Talarmin, P. Dubrous, 'Antibiotic Sensitivity to Epidemic Strains of *Vibrio cholerae* and *Shigella dysenteriae I* Isolated in Refugee Camps in Zaire', *Médecine Tropicale (Marseilles)*, 55 (1995) pp. 172–7; C. Paquet, P. Leborgne, A. Sasse, F. Varaine, 'An Outbreak of Shigella Dysenteriae Type 1 in a Refugee Camp in Rwanda', *Sante*, 5 (1995) pp. 181–4.

24 P. Shears, A. M. Berry, R. Murphy, M. A. Nabil, 'Epidemiological Assessment of the Health and Nutrition of Ethiopian Refugees in Emergency Camps in Sudan, 1985', *British Medical Journal*, 295 (1987) pp. 314–18.

25 M. J. Toole, R. J. Steketee, R. J. Waldman and P. Nieburg, 'Measles Prevention and Control in Emergency Settings', *Bulletin of the World Health Organisation*, 67 (1989) pp. 381–8.

26 'Public Health Impact of Rwandan Refugee Crisis', op. cit.; M. J. Toole and R. J. Waldman, 'Refugees and Displaced Persons: War, Hunger, and Public Health', *JAMA*, 270 (1993) pp. 600–5.

27 M. J. Toole and R. J. Waldman, 'The Public Health Aspects of Complex Emergencies and Refugee Situations', *Annual Review of Public Health, 1997*.

28 D. Wolday, T. Kibreab, D. Bukenya, R. Hodes, 'Sensitivity of Plasmodium Falciparum in vivo to Chloroquine and Pyrimethamine-Sulfadoxine in a Refugee Camp in Zaire', *Transcriptions of the Royal Society for Tropical Medicine and Hygiene*, 89 (1995) pp. 654–6; F. Nosten, F. Kuile, T. Chongsuphajaisiddhi, C. Luxemburger, H. K. Webster, M. Edstein, L. Phaipun, K. L. Thew and N. J. White, 'Mefloquine Resistant Falciparum Malaria on the Thai-Burmese Border', *Lancet*, 337 (1991) pp. 1140–3.

29 C. Beadle, S. L. Hoffman, 'History of Malaria in the United States Naval Forces at War: World War I through the Vietnam Conflict', *Clinical Infectious Diseases*, 16 (1993) pp. 320–9; V. P. Sergiev, A. M. Baranova, V. S. Orlov, L. G. Mihajlov, R. L. Kouznetsov, N. I. Neujmin, L. P. Arsenieva, M. A. Shahova, L. A. Glagoleva and M. M. Osipova, 'Importation of Malaria into the USSR from Afghanistan, 1981–9', *Bulletin of the World Health Organization*, 71 (1993) pp. 385–8.

30 J. Y. Riou, S. Djibo, L. Sangare, J. P. Lombart, P. Fagot, J. P. Chippaux and M. Guibourdenche, 'A Predictable Comeback: the Second Pandemic of Infections Caused by Neisseria Meningitidis Serogroup A subgroup III in Africa, 1995', *Bulletin of the World Health Organisation*, 74(2) (1996) pp. 181–7; M. Guibourdenche, D. A. Caugant, V. Herve, J. M. Debonne, C. Lanckriet, M. Merlin, C. Mathiot, J. B. Roungou, G. Martet and J. Y. Riou, 'Characteristics of Serogroup A Neisseria Meningitidis Strains Isolated in the Central African Republic in February 1992', *European Journal of Clinical Microbiology and Infectious Diseases*, 13(2) (1994) pp. 174–7.

31 P. S. Moore, M. J. Toole et al., 'Surveillance and Control of Meningococcal Meningitis Epidemics in Refugee Populations', *Bulletin of the World Health Organisation*, 68 (1990) pp. 587–96.

32 E. Haelterman, M. Boelaert, C. Suetens, L. Blok, M. Henkens and M. J. Toole, 'Impact of a Mass Vaccination Campaign against a Meningitis Epidemic in a Refugee Camp', *Tropical Medicine and International Health*, 1 (1996) pp. 385–92.

33 'Famine-Affected, Refugee and Displaced Populations', op. cit.

34 E. E. Mast, L. B. Polish, M. O. Favorov et al., 'Hepatitis E among Refugees in Kenya: Minimal Apparent Person-to-Person Transmission, Evidence for Age-Dependent Disease Expression, and New Serological Assays', in K. Kishioka, H. Suzuki, S. Mishiro and T. Oda (eds), *Viral Hepatitis and Liver Disease* (Tokyo: Springer-Verlag, 1994) pp. 375–8.

35 K. Bile, A. Isse, O. Mohamud et al., 'Contrasting Roles of Rivers and Wells as Sources of Drinking Water on Attack and Fatality Rates in a Hepatitis E Epidemic in Somalia', *American Journal of Tropical Medicine and Hygiene*, 51(4) (1994) pp. 466–74.

36 M. J. Toole, S. Galson, W. Brady, 'Are War and Public Health Compatible?' *Lancet*, 341 (1993) pp. 935–8.

37 P. Sudre, 'Tuberculosis Control in Somalia', World Health Organization EM/ TUB/180/E/R/5.93 (Geneva, May 1993).

38 R. G. Barr, R. Menzies, 'The Effect of War on Tuberculosis: Results of a Tuberculin Survey among Displaced Persons in El Salvador and a Review of the Literature', *Tuberculosis and Lung Disease*, 75 (1994) pp. 251–9.

39 'Famine-Affected, Refugee and Displaced Populations', op. cit.

40 C. R. MacIntyre, B. Dwyer and J. A. Streeton, 'The Epidemiology of Tuberculosis in Victoria', *Medical Journal of Australia*, 159 (1993) pp. 672–7.

41 M. R. Smallman-Raynor and A. D. Cliff, 'Civil War and the Spread of AIDS in Central Africa', *Epidemiology of Infections*, 107 (1991) pp. 69–80.

42 Unpublished data, B. Brady, Centers for Disease Control and Prevention, Atlanta, 1992.

43 S. Swiss, J. Giller, 'Rape as a Crime of War', *JAMA*, 270 (1993) pp. 612–15.

44 W. A. Perea, T. Ancelle, A. Moren, M. Nagelkerke and E. Sondorp, 'Visceral Leishmaniasis in Southern Sudan', *Transcriptions of the Royal Society of Tropical Medicine and Hygiene*, 85 (1991) pp. 48–53.

45 E. E. Zijlstra, M. S. Ali, A. M. el-Hassan, I. A. el-Toum, M. Satti, H. W. Ghali, E. Sondorp and A. Winkler, *Transcriptions of the Royal Society of Tropical Medicine and Hygiene*, 85 (1991) pp. 365–9.

46 A. Hailu, N. Berhe and H. Yeneheh, 'Visceral Leishmaniasis in Gambela, Western Ethiopia', *Ethiopian Medical Journal*, 34 (1996) pp. 33–42.

47 H. Wilde, J. Pornsilapatip, T. Sokly and S. Thee, 'Murine and Scrub Typhus at Thai-Kampuchean Border Displaced Persons Camps', *Tropical Geography and Medicine*, 43 (1991) pp 363–9.

48 'Famine-Affected, Refugee and Displaced Populations', op. cit.

49 World Health Organization, 'Guidelines for Cholera Control', WHO/CDD/ SER/80.4 Rev 2 (Geneva, 1990).

50 'Famine-Affected, Refugee and Displaced Populations', op. cit.

51 J. C. Desenclos (ed.), *Clinical Guidelines: Diagnostic and Treatment Manual.* Second Edition (Paris: Médecins Sans Frontières, 1992); C. Mears and S. Chowdhury (eds), *Health Care for Refugees and Displaced People* (Oxford: Oxfam,1994).

52 World Health Organization, 'The Treatment of Acute Diarrhoea', WHO/ CDD/SER/80.2. Rev.1 (Geneva, 1984).

7
The HIV/AIDS Epidemic: Public Policies and Possessive Individualism

Renée Danziger

Faced with the challenge of HIV and AIDS, policy-makers have by and large drawn on public health traditions which emphasize individual autonomy and personal choice in preference to those which are based on universalism and compulsion. In some instances, policy-makers have broken with tradition altogether by prioritizing individual rights to an extent previously unknown in a public health context. This chapter explores three policy areas in which this has occurred. The novelty of the policies under consideration is attributed here to the peculiar clinical, epidemiological and demographic characteristics of HIV and AIDS, combined with an ideological context characterized by possessive individualism within which the policies have evolved.

In the early 1980s the US Centers for Disease Control (CDC) observed in previously healthy homosexual men diseases which had hitherto only occurred in people with severely compromised immune systems. In June 1981 five cases of pneumocystis carinii pneumonia were reported in young homosexual men in Los Angeles, and the next month it was disclosed that 26 young homosexual men had earlier been diagnosed with Kaposi's sarcoma, a rare form of cancer which had until then been associated with elderly Americans.[1] At the time, nobody could have foretold that these were the first signs of a new epidemic which would cost the world hundreds of thousands of lives.

1983 marks a watershed in the history of the epidemic, for this was the year that the human immunodeficiency virus (HIV) was identified as the virus that causes AIDS. Within a relatively short time it was established that HIV transmission could occur through sexual intercourse (both anal and vaginal); receipt of infected blood (or blood products)

130

Table 7.1 Estimated number of people with HIV infection (1996)

North America	750 000
Caribbean	270 000
Latin America	1 300 000
Western Europe	510 000
North Africa and Middle East	200 000
Sub-Saharan Africa	14 000 000
Eastern Europe and Central Asia	50 000
South and South-East Asia	5 200 000
East Asia and Pacific	100 000
Australasia	13 000
Global total	22 600 000

Source: UNAIDS

through transfusion or through the use of contaminated injecting equipment; and from mother to child *in utero*, at birth or through breast milk. The current cumulative total number of reported AIDS cases worldwide stands at 8.4 million and there are an additional estimated 22.6 million cases of HIV infection. With new infections occurring at an increasing rate (currently approximately 10 000 a day), AIDS cases would continue to escalate over the coming years *even if* transmission were to stop overnight.[2]

AIDS is not a single disease as such, but rather a 'syndrome'. People with AIDS may suffer from a variety of different medical conditions, including cancers and infections, to which they are vulnerable as a result of their reduced immunological defences caused by infection with HIV.

Although AIDS is widely viewed as ultimately fatal, the length of time that a person can live with AIDS varies greatly from one individual to another. Important factors influencing longevity include health status prior to infection with HIV, and also access to healthy foods, appropriate shelter, psychosocial support and treatments for opportunistic infections. In addition, increasing evidence suggests that combination therapies involving protease inhibitors may significantly prolong life with HIV and AIDS.[3] However, as these therapies cost an estimated US$10 000–$20 000 per person per year, they remain far beyond the means of the vast majority of people with AIDS, 90 per cent of whom live in developing countries.[4]

As HIV has spread silently around the world, growing numbers of people have been touched by the epidemic, either directly through HIV infection and AIDS, or through the infection of family members, lovers, friends, colleagues, acquaintances or patients. For many of those affected by the epidemic, HIV/AIDS came to represent the single greatest public health challenge of the late twentieth century. But for the many more who have yet to feel the effects of HIV/AIDS, there is surprise and often resentment at the amount of time, energy and most of all the resources which have been invested in the control of the epidemic. While more than 100 000 people die annually as a result of AIDS, one million die every year from malaria, three million from tuberculosis, four million from diarrhoeal disease, five million from cancer, and 12 million from heart and other cardiovascular diseases.[5] Why have so many people devoted so much attention to addressing HIV/AIDS?

One reason is that HIV is spreading much faster than malaria, tuberculosis, heart disease and cancer, which adds urgency to efforts to reduce HIV transmission.

Achieving a reduction is complicated, however, because of the ways in which HIV is transmitted. Globally the most common route of transmission is sexual contact: in most developing countries it is heterosexual contact, while in many developed countries it is homosexual contact. In a few countries, mainly in southern Europe, sexual transmission has come second to transmission via blood among injecting drug users who have shared contaminated injecting equipment.

In the absence of a vaccine, efforts to stop the spread of the virus have concentrated on changing sexual and drug using behaviours. Influencing such intimate and often covert activities represents a major challenge to public health professionals.

The modes of transmission are important for another reason. Most of the people who have been infected by HIV, or who are at risk of infection, have been or are sexually active, and in a smaller number of cases they self-inject drugs. These are typically people between 20 and 40 years old: society's most economically productive and socially active individuals. This contrasts with many other major diseases which tend to affect mainly either the very young, or the very old.[6]

The nature of HIV infection also sets the epidemic apart from others. A person can be infected with the virus and yet remain healthy for many years before developing symptoms of AIDS. HIV prevention workers have had to take into account the possibility that many people may be unaware of their infection and unwittingly pass it on to other people. New preventive strategies have been required to respond to this distinctive feature of the epidemic.

Awareness of these unique clinical, epidemiological and demographic features of HIV and AIDS helps in understanding the innovative quality of some of the policy responses associated with the epidemic. In addition, one also needs to consider the peculiar interplay between these features on the one hand, and the social context in which HIV/AIDS policies have been developed on the other.

The late twentieth century was marked in many parts of the world by the pre-eminence of a neoliberal democratic ideology – an ideology which elevates the rights and interests of individuals *qua* individuals over and above those of collectivities. Although this ideology is most clearly articulated and widely embraced in the developed world, some have identified neoliberalism as a global phenomenon.[7] C. B. MacPherson argues cogently that contemporary ideas of (neo)liberal democracy are rooted in seventeenth-century individualism, which is itself characterized by a possessive quality (hence MacPherson's 'political theory of possessive individualism').

Its possessive quality is found in its conception of the individual as essentially the proprietor of his own person or capacities, owing nothing to society for them. The individual was seen neither as a moral whole, nor as part of a larger social whole, but as an owner of himself. ... The individual, it was thought, is free inasmuch as he is proprietor of his person and capacities. The human essence is freedom from dependence on the wills of others, and freedom is a function of possession. Society becomes a lot of free equal individuals related to each other as proprietors of their own capacities and of what they have acquired by this exercise. Society consists of relations of exchange between proprietors.[8]

The pivotal role of the individual as 'proprietor of his own person' is perhaps most clearly expressed in the principles of neoliberal economics, according to which each individual relies on his or her own properties (education, skills, and so on) in order to secure gains (jobs, salary, benefits, and so forth) within a (relatively) free market. The state's responsibility is to ensure that every individual can exercise his or her right to enter this marketplace, 'which consists of relations of exchange between proprietors'.

The values of possessive individualism are equally reflected in policies which have been developed in response to HIV and AIDS. Policy-makers have by and large eschewed collective and compulsory measures and drawn instead on public health traditions which have stressed individual autonomy and personal choice. In some instances they have broken with tradition altogether by placing protection of individual rights on a par with (or even above) the protection of the public health.

This chapter will explore three areas in which this appears to have occurred: (1) the linkage between HIV prevention and human rights protection, whereby human rights protection has become as much of a priority as HIV prevention; (2) the emphasis on individual consent rather than on more universal approaches to testing for HIV infection; and (3) the newly acquired relative autonomy of individual patients in determining the course of their medical treatment. Although these policy areas have unarguably had most relevance for developed countries, many of the debates surrounding them have also influenced to differing extents the policy agendas of many developing countries.

HIV prevention and human rights protection

Placing human rights on the AIDS agenda

The relationship between human rights protection on the one hand, and disease prevention on the other has never been made so explicit as in the case of HIV/AIDS. One of the reasons that human rights (and civil liberties) have featured so prominently is that HIV is transmitted mainly through deeply private and, in some contexts, even illegal behaviours. State interference in these extremely personal aspects of life, even in the supposed interests of disease control, is anathema for many people who have vociferously defended personal liberties.

Another reason concerns the social and historical context in which the epidemic emerged. HIV/AIDS appeared in the USA and certain other developed countries shortly after gay rights organizations had achieved a degree of political influence. As awareness of the meaning of HIV for the gay community grew, some of these pre-existing groups mobilized swiftly in order to ensure that governments did not infringe upon newly won rights in their efforts to control the spread of the virus. Although over time HIV also affected large numbers of drug users, haemophiliacs and women, in the main it was gay organizations which were most instrumental in shaping the HIV prevention agenda, and ensuring that human rights protection was high up on that agenda. This is largely because, unlike other groups affected by the epidemic, they were already organized, politicized, and familiar with the discourse of human rights.[9]

There is another historical factor which helps to explain the unprecedented prominence of human rights in the context of disease prevention. AIDS appeared at a time when the language of human rights was common parlance. In the 1970s and 80s an international consensus had developed, in which governments were widely considered to be legitimate to the extent that they were seen to respect and protect the human rights of their constituents.[10] It is beyond the scope of this chapter to consider where and how this consensus arose. What is relevant here is that in the context of this widely embraced ideology, which promoted the rights of individuals *qua* individuals, it was often difficult for policymakers to refute claims that the HIV/AIDS agenda should incorporate effective human rights protection.

One of the most remarkable aspects of AIDS policy in this connection is that human rights protection often came to assume *as high* a priority as HIV prevention itself. Voluntarism and protection of individual liberties were often upheld not simply because they were believed to be effective in HIV prevention, but because they were regarded as inherently valuable. Thus, in the view of at least one influential commentator, even if particular public health measures appear to achieve the aim of preventing the spread of disease, 'the imperatives of prevention, however important, are not the only values to be considered in the struggle against AIDS'.[11]

In the early years of the epidemic, it was chiefly the non-governmental organizations (NGOs) working on HIV/AIDS in developed countries which championed the 'human rights approach' to HIV prevention and control. Much less was heard about human rights and AIDS from government agencies. Yet within a relatively short time, governments around the world were speaking about a link between HIV prevention and human rights protection, and in many cases were incorporating this in their national AIDS programmes. How did this transformation occur?

While AIDS NGOs consistently lobbied their governments, at the same time the World Health Organization's Global Programme on AIDS (WHO/GPA) also worked to ensure that governments protected human rights in the context of HIV/AIDS.

WHO was in an ideal position to do this. It established its AIDS Programme in 1986, and a year later the Programme was mandated by the United Nations General Assembly to coordinate and provide leadership to AIDS prevention and care programmes around the world. By 1990 the Programme employed over 100 staff, had a budget of US$100 million, and had already provided collaborative assistance to 159 countries around the world.[12]

The Programme was led and staffed by individuals who were themselves committed to the principles of civil liberties and individual human rights. Because of both the remit and the resources available to WHO/GPA, these individuals had a unique opportunity to promote the language and values of human rights in AIDS programmes around the world. This was carried out at three levels.

First, WHO/GPA brought the issue of human rights to the highest levels of health policy-making including the World Summit of Ministers of Health in 1987 and the World Health Assembly in 1988. Second, WHO/GPA used a carrot-and-stick approach to ensure that human rights protection was integrated in the work of national AIDS programmes and NGOs. GPA refused to fund country activities which threatened human rights, while providing technical and financial support to projects which sought expressly to address human rights concerns in the context of HIV/AIDS.[13]

Third, and perhaps most influentially, WHO/GPA employed a combination of persuasion and pressure to intervene on specific human rights issues. A notable example of this relates to the issue of HIV and international travel. In 1988 WHO, then a co-sponsor of the Sixth International Conference on AIDS, successfully opposed the siting of the Conference in San Francisco on grounds that US federal regulations were discriminatory because they prohibited foreigners with HIV infection from entering the country for more than a short period. The impact of this manoeuvre (combined with an expert meeting convened earlier by WHO/GPA to look at AIDS and travel) was considerable, and was widely believed to have 'contributed to preventing an impending wave of restrictive legislation'.[14]

Prevention of HIV/AIDS-related discrimination

The human rights issue which WHO/GPA was most actively concerned with was the principle of non-discrimination in the context of HIV/AIDS. Two reasons were given for avoiding discrimination on the basis of HIV. First, discrimination was regarded as an unjustifiable attack on the human rights and dignity enshrined in the Universal Declaration of Human Rights.[15] Whereas previously disease control had always been discussed chiefly in terms of what works (which might in some cases include voluntarism, confidentiality and a non-stigmatizing approach),[16] in the case of AIDS considerable concern was expressed about the need to protect human rights as an end in itself.

A second reason given for avoiding HIV/AIDS related discrimination was grounded in public health concerns. The argument most frequently articulated in this connection was that:

if HIV infection or suspicion of HIV infection, leads to stigmatisation and discrimination (e.g. loss of employment, forced separation from family, loss of education or housing), persons already HIV-infected and those who are concerned they may be infected will actively avoid detection and contact with health and social services will be lost. Those needing information, education, counselling or other support services would be 'driven underground'. The person who fears he or she may be infected would be reluctant to seek assistance out of fear of being reported – with severe personal consequences. The net result would be to seriously jeopardise educational outreach and thereby exacerbate the difficulty of preventing HIV infection.[17]

Most efforts to reduce HIV/AIDS-related discrimination have been based either on educational programmes or legislation – chiefly the former. Posters in Uganda encourage the public to 'Care for people with AIDS'; the Brazilian AIDS campaign has urged solidarity; and in California, a poster with a drawing of a child which reads: 'I have AIDS. Please hug me – I can't make you sick' has been reproduced all around the world.[18] Other educational efforts include training programmes to heighten awareness of HIV/AIDS discrimination. The AIDS and Law Project in South Africa, for example, provides training to prison officers and prisoners to help prevent HIV/AIDS-related discrimination within the prison service.[19] In Tunisia, a workshop was held for doctors and nurses from 13 countries in the region to examine clinical management, nursing and counselling from the point of view of avoiding HIV/AIDS-related discrimination.

There are more cases of information and education being used as strategies to reduce HIV/AIDS related discrimination than anti-discrimination legislation, although some notable examples of legislative strategies for reducing discrimination can be found. In the former Soviet Union, the Law on Prevention of AIDS of 23 April 1990 states that dismissal from work, refusal of admission to educational establishments, and 'the restriction of other rights' on the grounds of HIV infection 'shall be prohibited'. The Japanese AIDS Prevention Law of 23 December 1988 declares (somewhat ambiguously) that the authorities 'shall give consideration to protecting the human rights of AIDS patients'.[20] In New York City, the Commission on Human Rights combines education with litigation to pre-empt or reverse discrimination against people on the grounds of HIV status.[21]

Few diseases, if any, have been so closely identified with human rights concerns as HIV/AIDS. While previous diseases, including syphilis and gonorrhoea, had sometimes been treated on a voluntary rather than compulsory basis, this has been because the voluntarist approach was believed to be more effective in public health terms. Conversely, in the case of HIV prevention, human rights protection has been seen as inherently important and has become non-negotiable on many AIDS agendas.

Yet notwithstanding the formal agendas, discrimination continues to occur both at the level of civil society and the state. Examples are numerous: the firebombing of a shelter for children of HIV-infected parents; the stigmatization of women whose husbands die of AIDS; refusal to employ people because they are known or presumed to be HIV infected; the eviction of families from their homes; and refusing entry into a country because of HIV infection. The list is all but endless.

Individual versus universal approaches to name-linked HIV testing

All people who are identified as HIV positive risk discrimination, and it has been partly in order to avert experiences of discrimination that so many AIDS activists and public health workers have opposed routine or mandatory name-linked testing for HIV.

HIV testing first became available in 1985. At the time it was widely seen as a major breakthrough for HIV prevention. Not least, the ability to detect HIV antibodies in blood made it technically possible to ensure safe blood supplies. However, it still remains unclear whether name-linked HIV testing brings about the behaviour changes which are necessary to prevent HIV transmission via sexual contact or injecting drug use.

The ambiguity surrounding the relationship between HIV testing and risk reduction derives chiefly from methodological obstacles to the attribution of causality.[22] Such studies as have been conducted on the subject have produced very mixed and sometimes contradictory results.[23]

Given the uncertainty about the preventive role of HIV testing, many have argued that mandatory testing constitutes an unjustified invasion of individuals' privacy. This is especially the case in view of the fact that until very recently, the individual who was being tested had little to gain from the experience. On the contrary, a negative test result could lead to a false sense of security and then increased risk behaviours, while a positive result would bring with it intense psychosocial pain and suffering as well as the risk of discrimination by those who found out about the test result. The economic cost of widespread testing has served as a further major disincentive to advocating widespread testing for HIV, particularly in many developing countries, where health budgets often do not cover the basic needs of the population.[24]

In view of the above considerations, and in keeping with the values of possessive individualism, it has been argued that the only circumstances under which testing should take place would be where the individual had freely consented to being tested, having first been informed of the short- and long-term implications of HIV testing.[25]

There have, however, been a relatively small number of public health authorities that have rejected this paradigm, and insisted instead that HIV be addressed in the same, more universal, manner as many other infectious diseases, namely by routinely – and if necessary compulsorily – testing populations with a view to identifying those who are infected and taking whatever steps are possible to prevent them from infecting others. What these steps might be depends on the context. In Hungary, for example, where testing is mandatory for certain groups including sexually transmitted disease patients, people who are identified as HIV positive are required to return to the authorities for counselling (and treatment if appropriate) every three months, at which time they are reminded of the need to prevent onward transmission of the virus.[26] In Cuba, mass screening of the population has been accompanied by a comprehensive programme of education and care during which HIV positive people are temporarily removed from the wider society and housed in one of 12 AIDS residential communities (sanatoriums) at which patients are given medical treatment, counselling and advice about avoiding onward transmission of HIV.[27]

Even some of the most committed supporters of voluntarism have been obliged to admit that 'Cuban policy will certainly limit the toll of HIV infection in Cuba dramatically'.[28] Yet in spite of this, they have maintained that such policies are at best questionable because of the infringement of individual liberties which is involved.

Voluntarists have argued that HIV should *not* be treated like those diseases (such as syphilis) which have been (and still are) routinely screened for. They point out that, unlike many such diseases, HIV cannot be cured or treated and consequently there are no means by which to *ensure* that the individual will not pass on the infection. Moreover – and possibly more importantly – the HIV-infected individual has until now reaped little benefit from being tested and identified as HIV positive. As the principles of possessive individualism dictate, individuals are the proprietors of their own persons, and should therefore be the ones to decide whether or not to be tested.

Although there are pockets of resistance (such as Cuba and Hungary), in the main the approach taken to HIV prevention in general and HIV testing more specifically has been firmly rooted in these liberal, voluntarist convictions. One commentator was moved to write of an 'uncanny consensus' which now exists around the world regarding the caveat that the AIDS epidemic should not be compared to other, earlier epidemics (whether of influenza, tuberculosis, or syphilis); the insistence that AIDS be treated as a 'special case'; and the acceptance of individually-oriented education programs as the only acceptable form of AIDS prevention.[29]

How can the apparent consensus around voluntarism in HIV prevention be accounted for? At one level, it could be argued that it reflects the internal coherence of the public health arguments advanced by committed voluntarists. The skill with which these arguments have been put forward, by NGOs, public health officials, and WHO among others, has also undoubtedly helped to ensure the depth and breadth of the consensus. But perhaps most importantly, the arguments appear almost irrefutable in a social context wherein the sovereign value of individual rights, personal choice and the unfettered pursuit of one's own interests is considered to be virtually incontrovertible. Those who challenge this framework of understanding form a small minority which is on the political margins.

The debate around HIV testing will without doubt change over the coming months and years, as biomedical advances bring forward the possibility of treating HIV and preventing AIDS.[30] As treatments become increasingly effective, discussion will focus more on the issue of the *cost* of treating HIV. This raises broader questions about who should have access to HIV drugs and through which procedures. Some of these questions are considered below.

The role of the patient in determining medical care and treatment

A unique feature of the HIV/AIDS epidemic has been the role played by the people most directly affected by it in determining the availability and accessibility of medical care and treatment. This has been most notably the case in the USA, and to a lesser extent in Europe. In this chapter, the focus will be on developments in the US, because it was here that AIDS had its greatest impact on the drug regulation process.

In the United States, the Food and Drug Administration (FDA) holds statutory authority for regulating and overseeing the processes of drug manufacture, marketing, promotion and testing. Throughout the 1960s and 1970s, the overriding aim of the FDA in discharging these duties was to ensure that only 'safe' drugs were approved and marketed in the US, 'leaving to others like the National Institutes of Health (NIH), to worry about curing disease'.[31]

The second – and some would say secondary – concern of the FDA was in establishing the efficacy of a drug before approving it for public use. Efficacy was determined through clearly defined procedures, namely through multiple controlled clinical trials. Controlled clinical trials often took a long time to carry out but despite this – and perhaps partly because of this – controlled trials became the gold standard for providing 'scientific proof' of the efficacy of drugs.

Through rigorous application of its strict criteria of safety and efficacy, the FDA not only regulated the flood of new drug applications, but it also assumed the role of guardian of the public well-being. This essentially paternalistic role reflected the social welfare approach which was taken towards public policy more generally at the time. The FDA was understood to be responsible for deciding whether a particular drug should and could be released onto the market for popular consumption. The relationship between drug companies, the FDA and the consumer which was thus established was to undergo profound change with the advent of the AIDS epidemic in the 1980s.

During the 1980s and 1990s, rising numbers of people with HIV and AIDS, and organizations representing them, have assumed responsibility both for informing themselves about all aspects of experimental and approved AIDS treatments, and for taking action where this has been deemed necessary to reform the drug regulation process. This in itself marks something of a reversal from the 'structural iatrogenesis' of the 1960s and 1970s when patients appeared content to allow medical professionals to make decisions on their behalf.[32]

The turnaround in attitude witnessed in the 1980s can be explained partly by the keen determination to live of many people with AIDS, who were often less than forty years old. In addition, the rising anger, frustration and despair at what was perceived as an unacceptably slow policy response to HIV/AIDS by political leaders spilled over into dissatisfaction with the drug regulation process. The articulation of this dissatisfaction, and the assertion of individual choices and rights regarding medical treatment can also be understood within the context of possessive individualism according to which individuals are relatively autonomous beings, with rights and responsibilities for their own well-being. It is in this context that AIDS activists challenged traditional practices on drug regulation.

Probably the most important innovation achieved by AIDS activists and their allies in this connection concerned the changes introduced in the 'gold standard' design of clinical trials. Until the 1980s, proof of a drug's efficacy could only be established through a series of controlled trials, in which the drug was given to one group of patients and withheld from a comparable group of patients who were given a placebo instead. To enhance the reliability of the trial, double blinding was used, so that neither the patients nor their doctors knew whether it was the drug or the placebo which was being administered.

Many AIDS activists objected to the requisite use of double-blinded controls for experimental AIDS drugs. First, it was argued that the system of testing new drugs 'should not deny individuals the right to choose their own therapeutic options simply because scientists need controls in order to determine by their own canons of evidence what works best'.[33] Many also began to question the paternalist role of the FDA, and to suggest that people with AIDS were well equipped to understand and decide on issues concerning their own treatment. A further objection was raised to the prevailing system of proving the efficacy of a drug. Many activists argued that the administration of placebos in the interests of scientific progress was unethical, when there was a possibility that the alternative – namely administration of the experimental drug – could save or prolong a person's life.

AIDS activists organized themselves around these issues and informed themselves extensively about the health implications of different therapeutic treatments which were being developed by pharmaceutical companies. One of the most prominent and powerful organizations to emerge out of this was the AIDS Coalition to Unleash Power (ACT UP), which was established in 1987. Through aggressive lobbying and advocacy ACT UP and its allies helped to bring forward the availability of a drug prior to completion of all clinical trials.

The first drug widely thought to slow down the progression of HIV/AIDS was zidovudine (AZT). After pressure by AIDS activists, AZT became available, albeit on a limited basis, *before* it was finally approved for marketing by the FDA. A few years later, more than 30 000 people were treated with dideoxynosine (ddI) while clinical trials were still under way and before the drug had been approved for marketing.[34]

In addition to bringing forward the work of the FDA, AIDS activists brought about change in another area, namely in the development of Community Research Initiatives (CRIs). The first of these came into being in 1986, with the establishment of the New York Community Research Initiative. This was a grassroots initiative by the People With AIDS Coalition, in collaboration with a number of clinicians and practitioners. CRIs, initially a uniquely American phenomenon, but now in existence in Britain, aimed at recruiting people into experimental drug programmes in which a major aim was the well-being of the people involved in the experiment. They sought to reverse the existing approach of the FDA and its scientific allies in which 'the drug researcher is not primarily concerned with providing optimal care for individual subjects',[35] but rather with establishing 'evidence' of the safety and efficacy of a drug for *future* use.

Thus, for example, the CRIs ensured that participants in experimental drug programmes received the necessary treatments for any opportunistic infections they might acquire, even at the risk of impairing the scientific rigour of the experiment and setting back progress.

The impact which people with HIV and AIDS have had on drug regulation is important, not only because of direct consequences for people with HIV and AIDS, but also for wider reasons. For better or worse, people with AIDS successfully challenged the moral and political authority of the FDA and its *modus operandi*, and raised important questions about the epistemological foundations of modern bio-medicine. In keeping with an ethic of possessive individualism, they demanded a role in the decision-making process rather than allowing an established paternalistic authority to make decisions on their behalf.

Conclusions

When future historians of medicine come to examine the development of HIV/AIDS, they will undoubtedly devote much attention to the immense biomedical challenge presented by the HIV virus. What may be even more striking than this, however, are the social and political dimensions of the epidemic.

For the first time, preventing the spread of an infectious disease has been treated as both a public health responsibility and a human rights concern. Whereas voluntarism may have featured in previous public health responses,[36] in the case of AIDS the emphasis placed on voluntarism and on human rights protection has been such that, in the words of Scheper-Hughes, '*AIDS was viewed as a crisis in human rights (that had some public health dimensions), rather than as a crisis in public health that had some important human rights dimensions.*'[37]

This chapter has attributed some of the key innovations associated with HIV/AIDS policies to the peculiar clinical, epidemiological and demographic characteristics of HIV and AIDS, coupled with the ideological context within which the policies have been developed, in which the individual is placed at the centre of the socio-political universe.

This is not to deny that concepts of community have played an important role in developing responses to HIV/AIDS. One of the most striking features of the epidemic has been the strength and visibility of solidarity

among some of the people affected by HIV and AIDS and those sym-
pathetic to them. The 'Red Ribbon' and the Names Project Quilt are two
well-known international symbols of this solidarity, and represent further
evidence of the unique character of the epidemic. However, although
solidarity plays a crucial social role, it is a quality which is neither promoted nor embodied in AIDS policies *per se*, which emphasize to a much
greater extent the interests, the rights, and the responsibilities of individuals *qua* individuals.

Probably the single most pressing issue facing AIDS policy-makers in
the coming years will be finding a means of ensuring that those in need
of medical treatment for HIV and AIDS can afford what is available.
Hopefully this problem will be addressed within a communitarian
framework, rather than being left to individuals to resolve, using whatever resources they have at their disposal as 'proprietors of their own
capacities'.

*Many thanks to Virginia Berridge, Susan Foster and Kelley Lee, all at the
London School of Hygiene and Tropical Medicine, for their extremely helpful
comments on an earlier draft of this chapter. This chapter was written with
financial support from the UK Economic and Social Research Council (ESRC).*

Notes

1 R. Bayer and D. Kirp, 'An Epidemic in Political and Policy Perspective', in
   D. Kirp and R. Bayer (eds), *AIDS in the Industrialised Democracies: Passions,
   Politics and Policies* (New Brunswick, NJ: Rutgers University Press, 1991).
2 *Lancet*, 'HIV: a War Still to be Won', (Editorial) *Lancet* 348 (1996) p. 1.
3 J. Montaner and M. T. Schechter, (1995) 'A Year of Transformation in HIV/
   AIDS', *Lancet* 346(supp.) (1995) p. 12; Scott Hammer, 'MO O1, Abstracts of
   the XIth International Conference on AIDS, Vancouver, July 7–12, 1996'.
4 M. Maddox 'The Lab', *Prospect*, 89 (1996).
5 Panos, *The Hidden Cost of AIDS: the Challenge of HIV to Development* (London:
   Panos Institute, 1992).
6 World Bank, *World Development Report: Investing in Health* (Washington, DC:
   World Bank, 1993).
7 K. Lee and A. Zwi, 'A Global Political Economy Approach to AIDS:
   Ideology, Interests and Implications', *New Political Economy* 1(3) (1996)
   pp. 355–73.
8 C. B. MacPherson, *The Political Theory of Possessive Individualism* (Oxford:
   Oxford University Press, 1962).
9 J. Ballard, 'Australia: Participation and Innovation in a Federal System', in
   D. L. Kirp and R. Bayer (eds), op. cit.; B. Henriksson, and H. Ytterberg, 'Sweden: the Power of the Moral(istic) Left', in D. L. Kirp and R. Bayer, op. cit.;
   M. Merson, 'Returning Home: Reflections on the USA's Response to the HIV/
   AIDS Epidemic', *Lancet*, 347 (1996) pp. 1673–6.
10 P. Jones, *Rights* (London: Macmillan, 1994).

11 R. Bayer, 'Controlling AIDS in Cuba: the Logic of Quarantine', *New England Journal of Medicine* 320(15) (1989) pp. 1022–4.

12 S. Collinson and K. Lee, 'What the United Nations Does on HIV/AIDS: From the WHO Global Programme on AIDS to UNAIDS', *UN and Health Briefing Note Number 5*, September 1996 (London School of Hygiene and Tropical Medicine).

13 J. Mann and K. Kay, (1991) 'Confronting the Pandemic: the World Health Organization's Global Programme on AIDS, 1986–1989', *AIDS* 5 (supp. 2) (1991) S221–S229.

14 Ibid.

15 United Nations, *Report of an International Consultation on AIDS and Human Rights*, Geneva 26–28 July 1989 (New York: United Nations, 1991).

16 V. Berridge, 'The History of AIDS', *AIDS* 7 (supp. 1) (1993) S243–S248.

17 J. Mann, 'AIDS, Discrimination and Public Health', Address presented at the IVth International Conference on AIDS, Stockholm, Sweden, 13 June 1988.

18 Panos, *The Third Epidemic: Repercussions of the Fear of AIDS* (London: Panos Institute, 1990).

19 AHRTAG, 'Rights and Respect', *AIDS Action*, no. 33, June–August 1996.

20 K. Tomasevski, K, 'The AIDS Pandemic and Human Rights', *Collected Courses of the Academy of European Law, Volume II, Book 2* (The Hague: Kluwer International, 1993) pp. 99–150.

21 New York Commission on Human Rights, *The Benefits and Limitations of AIDS Anti-Discrimination Legislation* (New York: City of New York Commission on Human Rights, 1991).

22 S. Beardsell, 'Should Wider HIV Testing be Encouraged on the Grounds of HIV Prevention?' *AIDS Care*, 6(1) (1994) pp. 5–19.

23 D. Higgins, C. Galavotti, K. R. O'Reilly et al., 'Evidence for the Effects of HIV Antibody Counselling and Testing on Risk Behaviours', *Journal of the American Medical Association* 266 (1991) pp. 2419–29; M. Horton, 'Bugs, Drugs and Placebos: the Opulence of Truth, or How to Make a Treatment Decision in an Epidemic', in E. Carter and S. Watney, *Taking Liberties* (London: Serpent's Tail, 1989).

24 R. Colebunders and P. Ndumben, 'Priorities for HIV Testing in Developing Countries?' *Lancet*, 342 (1993) pp. 601–2.

25 WHO, *Statement for the Consultation on Testing and Counselling for HIV Infection* (Geneva: World Health Organization, 16–18 November 1992).

26 R. Danziger, 'Compulsory Testing for HIV in Hungary', *Social Science and Medicine*, 43(8) (1996) pp. 1199–204.

27 N. Scheper-Hughes, 'An Essay: AIDS and the Social Body', *Social Science and Medicine*, 39(7) (1994) pp. 991–1003.

28 R. Bayer, 'Controlling AIDS in Cuba', op. cit.

29 Scheper-Hughes, 'An Essay', op. cit.

30 Scott Hammer, op. cit.; R. Danziger, 'An Epidemic Like Any Other? Rights and Responsibilities in HIV Prevention', *British Medical Journal*, 312 (1996) pp. 1083–4.

31 H. Edgar and D. J. Rothman, 'New Rules for New Drugs: the Challenge of AIDS to the Regulatory Process', in D. Nelkins, D. P. Willis and S. V. Parris (eds), *A Disease of Society: Cultural and Institutional Responses to AIDS* (Cambridge: Cambridge University Press, 1991).

32   I. Illich, *Medical Nemesis: the Expropriation of Health* (London: Calder & Boyers, 1975).
33   Edgar and Rothman, 'New Rules', op. cit.
34   N. Gilmore, 'The Impact of AIDS on Drug Availability and Accessibility', *AIDS* 5 (supp. 2) (1991) S253–S262.
35   Horton, 'Bugs, Drugs and Placebos', op. cit.
36   Berridge, 'The History of AIDS', op. cit.
37   Scheper-Hughes, 'An Essay', op. cit. (italics original).

8
Technological Change and Future Biological Warfare

Malcolm Dando

Introduction

In late April 1998 the *International Herald Tribune* ran a report of an exercise carried out with the aim of testing US capabilities to respond to a terrorist attack using biological weapons.[1] The report stated that capabilities were found to be very deficient, despite the considerable recent efforts to enhance them. The scenario for the table-top exercise was that 'terrorists spread a virus along the Mexican–American border, primarily in California and the Southwest', and, 'As the scenario unfolded, officials playing the role of state and local officials were quickly overwhelmed by a panicked population, thousands of whom were falling ill and dying.'

A major part of the problem was that the virus, initially taken to be smallpox, turned out to be 'a genetically engineered virus, a mix of the smallpox and Marburg viruses'. So, while smallpox vaccine was rushed in to immunize the people potentially at risk, they died of 'profuse bleeding and a high fever for which there was no cure'. The report noted the disagreement between respected scientists over whether such an attack was currently possible. The scenario was chosen as an extreme case which might reveal weaknesses in the civil defence system. Yet the report concluded that 'Experts tend to disagree on the plausibility of such high-technology threats. But most agree that the danger will grow and that such an attack, if successful, could be catastrophic'.

What are we to make of such an official exercise? Did it have a reasonable estimate of the kind of biological warfare agent that might be under development in offensive biological warfare programmes today and which the Biological and Toxin Weapons Convention (BTWC) Verification Protocol will have to be designed to restrict? The exercise was clearly designed as a serious test, but how extreme was the scenario? If this kind of agent is not available today but could be sometime in the future, how far in the future? Moreover, if this was not too extreme a threat scenario, or not too extreme in the near future, is this the only kind of new agent type we should be worried about? Could a smallpox-Marburg virus be but just one example of one type of a whole new range of threat possibilities? And if the development of modern biology and medicine is potentiating a vast range of new threat possibilities, could it not also be facilitating the considerable enhancement of defensive capabilities? How might the growth of offence and defence interact in the future?

In order to approach adequate answers to such questions we would need a model which incorporated, for example, consideration of the motives that might lead people to undertake offensive biological warfare programmes,[2] and of the different circumstances under which such programmes might flourish.[3] However, the focus here is on just one of the factors which might impact on the future of biological warfare – technological change. There are good reasons to think that state-level offensive military programmes will provide the cutting edge of weapon-system developments and that terrorists will follow the pattern set by the military. In this paper I shall consider only state-level offensive military programmes.

Do we need to consider such extreme threats?

Given the lethality of classical biological warfare agents,[4] it might reasonably be asked whether the exercise described earlier, and consequently any implications drawn from its results, has any credibility at all.

Smallpox virus belongs to the Poxviridae family of viruses. Smallpox (variola) virus is in the orthopoxvirus genus which also contains vaccinia virus, used for vaccinating against smallpox. Poxviruses are large viruses and can be seen, if suitably stained, with an ordinary light microscope. The orthopoxviruses are brick-shaped and about 230×270 nm in size. The genome of these viruses is made up of double-stranded DNA and is large enough to code for about 100 polypeptides. What is of particular interest here is that:

> genes of immunogenic proteins of rabies, influenza, HIV, and hepatitis have been cloned into the thymidine kinases (TK) locus of the genome of vaccinia virus. . . . The vaccinia virus genome is so large that its functions are not compromised by excision of a portion and reintroduction of a new section of nucleotides . . . [5]

Such possibilities have not gone unnoticed by those concerned with strengthening the BTWC. The UK's background paper on scientific and technological developments for the Fourth Review Conference in 1996 stated that:

> Genetically modified animal vaccines have also started to appear. An animal vaccine uses capripox virus as a vector to carry genes for Rinderpest virus antigens. This vaccine, which has the advantage of simultaneously protecting cattle against lumpy skin disease and Rinderpest, is currently undergoing trials in Kenya in closed conditions ... [6]

There are also suggestions of more malign activities in the literature. Marburg and Ebola viruses are classified in the family Filoviridae. These recently discovered 'emerging' viruses have small single-stranded RNA genomes. The severe illnesses they cause begin with a frontal headache and high fever and lead rapidly to serious bleeding from many body organs and death in a high proportion of those affected. According to Ken Alibek, the former member of the Soviet offensive biological warfare programme, one of his colleagues, Dr Nikolai Ustinov, died after accidentally injecting himself with Marburg virus. Then:

> They kept the Ustinov strain alive and continually replicating in the laboratories. ... They named the strain Variant U, after Ustinov, and they learnt how to mass-produce it. ... They dried Variant U, and processed it into an inhalable dust. The particles of Variant U were coated to protect them in air so that they would drift for many miles.[7]

The Variant U particles were found to be highly infective to monkeys and, again according to Alibek, in late 1991 the Marburg Variant U agent was on the verge of being a strategic/operational biological weapons agent for loading into MIRVed warheads.

Alibek also claims that the incapacitating VEE (Venezuelan Equine Encephalitis) virus was successfully spliced into the smallpox genome, in the Soviet programme in the early 1990s, without affecting the high lethality of the smallpox virus. More recently, he believes, the disease-causing parts of Ebola virus have been spliced into smallpox. Alibek has stated that 'As a weapon, the Ebolapox would give the haemorrhages and high mortality rate of Ebola virus ... plus the very high contagiousness of smallpox.'[8] The veracity of such claims has been questioned by both Russian and US scientists. However, it is sobering to recall that the Aum Shinrikyo sect were reported to be attempting to splice botulinum toxin genes into *E. coli* as part of efforts to develop their biological weapons of choice.[9]

The view, derived from the foregoing developments, that we should be concerned about future weaponry based on today's new biology is considerably reinforced by considering the growth of biology and its impact on offensive biological weapons programmes over the past century.

The impact of biology on twentieth-century military programmes

It is vital, given our current very relaxed stance towards infectious diseases, to understand just how recent our scientific knowledge and technological capabilities for control actually are. In the lead article in the 1989 *Annual Review of Microbiology* Harry Smith pointed out that:

> Today pathogenicity is a popular and exciting area of microbiology. Forty years ago, when I first became interested, studies on bacterial pathogenicity were moribund after their brilliant initial phase on toxins before the first world war. Those on viral pathogenicity had hardly started.[10]

The rapidity of advances in the 'Golden Age' of bacteriology at the end of the last century is still striking. The systematic nature of the work undertaken is evident from Robert Koch's postulates on what was necessary to prove the causal relationship between a micro-organism and a disease. He argued that:

- The micro-organism had to be present in every case of the disease;
- The micro-organism suspected of causing the disease had to be isolated and grown in a pure culture; and
- The disease had to occur when the isolated micro-organism was inoculated into a susceptible animal.

The new approach, driven by such conceptual and associated technical developments, allowed scientists to identify the bacterial agents causing many human and animal diseases (see Table 8.1). However, despite the recognition at the turn of the century that other, smaller, agents of disease – viruses – existed, it was not until the 1940s that technical advances 'opened what many regard as the "Golden Age of Virology" – the identification and isolation during the 1950s and 1960s of many viruses and their association with human diseases . . .'[11]

Table 8.1 Discovery of the bacteria causing some human and animal diseases

Date	Disease	Agent
1876	Anthrax	*Bacillus anthracis*
1880	Typhoid fever	*Salmonella typhi*
1882	Glanders	*Pseudomonas mallei*
1883	Cholera	*Vibrio cholerae*
1887	Malta (undulant) fever	*Brucella* spp.
1894	Plague	*Yersinia pestis*
1896	Botulism	*Clostridium botulinum*
1909	Rocky Mountain spotted fever	*Ricksettsia rickettsii*
1912	Tularemia	*Francisella tularensis*

Subsequently, of course, microbiology has become one of the integral components of the revolution in modern biotechnology and molecular biology. The impact of this tremendous increase in knowledge of biology, and its application in medicine, over the last 100 years can hardly be overestimated:

> The primary causes of [the] enormous mortality decline in the Western world lie in the unprecedented measure of control gained ... over infectious and parasitic diseases.... In contrast to the situation at the turn of the century, when infant mortality rates were of the order of 150 or more [per thousand] a number of western European countries today have single figure infant mortality rates ... [12]

It would be a considerable exception if this vast growth of organized knowledge had *not* also been applied to warfare.

In the historical record there are, of course, suggestions of the occasional use of biological warfare.[13] Well-known examples are the use of animal corpses to pollute water supplies, and the catapulting of diseased human corpses into besieged cities. However, it is difficult to produce conclusive proof of the deliberate use of disease until the distribution of smallpox-infected blankets by the British to North American Indians in the eighteenth century.[14] During the First World War, following the 'Golden Age' of bacteriology, it is now clear that *both* sides used pathogenic micro-organisms in attempts to sabotage valuable cavalry and draught animal stocks of opposition forces. The German sabotage campaign, at least in North America and Romania, is well documented,[15] and there is some evidence in the remaining French records of French activities.[16]

Table 8.2   French offensive biological warfare research 1919–1927*

Report of December 1922
'... laboratory trials were complete and enabled accurate information to be provided ...'
'... malaria and diphtheria could not be militarised ...'
'... rejected yellow fever and typhus because of the difficulties posed by the development of vectors for distribution'.
'... stressed the advantages offered by brucellosis (Maltese fever) which was easy to culture and had remarkable environmental resistance'.
'... possible to create artificially microbial clouds having all the physical properties of natural clouds and with an active duration of up to two hours. ... durability of microbial clouds and their infective capability depended on two factors: the dose and the relative humidity of the ambient air'.

* From Wheelis, 'Biological Sabotage' (see note 15).

Though the record of French activities between the wars is incomplete due to the occupation in the Second World War, it is clear that in the early 1920s they began a proper scientific study of the potential military use of biological weapons (Table 8.2). Although the 1925 Geneva Protocol had prohibited *first use* of biological weapons, offensive biological weapons programmes were not prohibited and a number of states are known to have undertaken such programmes prior to, and during, the Second World War. While numerous field trials (use) of biological warfare agents were carried out, and efforts made to weaponize agents in the massive Japanese programme,[17] the official British view at the end of the war was that: 'Japanese offensive BW was characterised by a curious mixture of foresight, energy, ingenuity, and at the same time, lack of imagination with surprisingly amateurish approaches to some aspects of the work.'[18] In particular, the British noted that the effective use of bombs loaded with biological agent was never achieved: 'the authorities ... disregarded any possible need for accumulation of quantitative data in cloud chambers preliminary to setting up field trials (indeed such chamber studies were never attempted).'

In the British offensive programme, under the direction of Paul Fildes, the doyen of British microbiology at that time, a very quantitative approach was adopted. Although Britain first developed an anti-animal capability by impregnating five million cattle cakes with anthrax spores, the main approach was based on careful evaluation of Britain's extensive experience with chemical weapons during the First World War. By November 1940,

> Fildes had determined that the most effective way would be to disseminate an aerosol of lung-retention sized particles from a liquid suspension of bacteria in a bursting munition such as a bomb delivered so that effective concentrations would be inhaled by anyone in the target area.[19]

It is perhaps also significant that while there were certainly studies of airborne particles in the last century, C. S. Cox, of the Chemical Defence Establishment at Porton Down in the UK, could write in 1987: 'That microorganisms can be spread by aerial transport through rooms, buildings, cities, continents and throughout the atmosphere, now is difficult to refute.'[20] He then immediately added: 'In contrast, at the turn of the century, the opposite view was held...and was still quite prevalent in the late 1930s.... This difference of opinion and the better understanding of today is largely due to the developing subject of Aerobiology.' The subject of aerobiology was launched, in part because greater aeroplane capabilities allowed better atmospheric sampling, in the early 1940s.[21]

British work concentrated on anthrax and, to a lesser extent, botulinal toxin and the British approach basically defined the main direction taken in other programmes for the rest of the century. British field trials quickly showed that biological weapons were much more potent than any chemical weapon, as has been repeatedly confirmed since. Before the end of the war British data were made available to the United States and Canada and a joint programme to produce an anthrax bomb was undertaken. While this project was not completed before the end of the war, some of the thinking behind the project[22] can be followed from official papers (Table 8.3).

The US offensive biological warfare programme persisted through a quarter of a century[23] and while it went through a number of phases (Table 8.4), the end result of this massive effort was the production and weaponization of a number of anti-personnel and anti-plant agents (Table 8.5). Clearly, as industrial production capabilities improved to meet the demand for antibiotics,[24] it became possible to produce the quantities of agent required in military programmes more easily. The potential operational use of biological weapons was also reconsidered so that instead of being thought of only as a retaliatory deterrent, as the official account notes: 'In 1956, a revised

Table 8.3 British view on the anthrax (N-bomb) project in late 1945*

N. is an A/C 500–lb cluster bomb containing 106 special bombs charged [with] anthrax spores. It is designed for strategic bombing as a reprisal. Detailed assessments have been considered . . .

(i) In general it has been thought that if 6 major German cities were attacked simultaneously by 2000 Lincolns armed with this weapon, 50% of the inhabitants who were exposed to the cloud of anthrax without respirators might be killed by inhalation, while many more might die through subsequent contamination of the skin . . . There is no danger of epidemic spread.

(ii) The terrain will be contaminated for years, and danger from skin infection should be great enough to enforce evacuation . . .

---

* From Gregory, *The Microbiology of the Atmosphere* (see note 21).

Table 8.4 The phases of the US Offensive Biological Warfare Programme*

Dates	Activity
1946–49	Research and planning years after World War II
1950–53	Expansion of the BW program during the Korean War
1954–58	Cold War years – reorganization of weapons and defense programs
1959–62	Limited war period – expanded research, development, testing and operational readiness
1963–68	Adaptation of the BW program to counter insurgencies – the Vietnam War years
1969–73	Disarmament and phase down

* From Joint Technical Warfare Committee, *Potentialities of Weapons* (see note 22).

BW/CW policy was formulated to the effect that the US would be prepared to use BW or CW in a general war to enhance military effectiveness.'[25]

As would be expected from the comparatively advanced state of bacteriology as against virology at the time, the US anti-personnel agent list was dominated (six to one) by bacteria and bacterial toxins. Again according to the official account:

Between 1954 and 1967 the facility [Pine Bluff Arsenal] produced the following biological agents and toxins: *Brucella suis*, *Pasturella tularensis*, Q fever rickettsia, Venezuelan Equine Encephalitis [VEE], *Bacillus anthracis*, botulinum toxin and staphylococcal enterotoxin. Bulk agents and antipersonnel munitions filled with those various agents and toxins were produced and stored . . .

Table 8.5 Some large-scale biological warfare agent production in the US*

Phase	Activity
1954–58	'... [Pine Bluff Arsenal] became operational in the spring of 1954 with the first production of *Brucella suis* (the causative agent of undulant fever). Large scale production of the lethal agent *Pasteurella tularensis* (tularemia) began a year later'.
1959–62	'... The advent of limited war and small scale conflict evoked a need for weapons which could assist in controlling conflict with minimum casualties. Controlled temporary incapacitation, therefore, became an ... objective, and CW and BW weapons offered the most promising technical possibilities. The BW program was then shifted to emphasise incapacitation.'
	'... The development of vaccines for Q fever and tularemia enabled development work on Q fever and tularemia to proceed to standardisation as BW agents ...'
1963–68	'In 1964 RDTE (Research, Development, Test, Evaluation) on enterotoxins from bacteria of the Staphylococcus group, which caused severe short term incapacitation ... had progressed to the point where development of weapon systems appeared feasible. As a result, work on this potential agent was accelerated ...'

* From Joint Technical Warfare Committee, *Potentialities of Weapons* (see note 22).

A number of anti-plant agents were also weaponized.

While we do not have a complete account of the Soviet programme, we do know that it continued after the US offensive programme was closed down and the Biological and Toxin Weapons Convention agreed in the early 1970s. Of course, the striking change that took place in biology in the 1970s was the demonstration of the possibility of recombinant DNA technology – genetic engineering.[26] This led to rapid progress, particularly as commercial possibilities were realized in medical applications (Table 8.6). Writing in 1986, Erhard Geissler noted, in a review mainly of US data, a shift in the kinds of organisms of interest to the military:

A comparison of the dates from the open literature ... shows that whereas in 1969 most of the organisms (20 out of 31) considered to be potential BW agents were *bacteria and fungi*, by 1983 *viruses* had become the majority of such agents (19 out of 22) ...[27]

He argued that the shift could have been caused by several factors including the greater ease of handling of dangerous viral agents made possible by genetic engineering:

Table 8.6   Some major events in the commercialisation of biotechnology*

Date	Event
1973	First cloning of a gene
1975	First hybridoma created
1981	First monoclonal antibody diagnostic kits approved for use in US
1982	First rDNA pharmaceutical product (human insulin) approved for use in US and UK
1983	First expression of a plant gene in a plant of a different species
1985	First US permit for experimental release of a genetically altered organism
1988	First US patent on an animal-transgenic mouse engineered to contain cancer genes
1990	First approval of human gene therapy clinical trial
1991	First approval of sale of genetically engineered biopesticide in US

* From Dando, 'New Developments in Biotechnology' (see note 24).

many of the viruses in the list of the potential BW agents have been previously considered as too dangerous or too difficult to handle for development as potential BW agents. However by 1983, the advent of genetic engineering techniques . . . had changed this situation . . .

In retrospect, therefore, it is hardly surprising that the Soviet programme of the 1980s involved weaponization of dangerous viral agents.[28] The potential misuse of genetic engineering, in the easier production of large amounts of toxins, was recognized at the Second Review Conference of the BTWC in 1986[29] and states became convinced that the Soviet programme involved the use of the new technology in additional ways after information from the first high-level defector, Dr Pasechnik, became available in the late 1980s: 'Natural plague is curable with antibiotics. After listening to Dr. Pasechnik, the British concluded that the Soviet Union had developed a genetically engineered strain of plague that was resistant to antibiotics . . . '.[30] The exact status of the programme appears to be a continuing official concern.

What we can see over the last century is a continuous process of military programmes developing on the back of growth in scientific knowledge. There have been three generations of offensive biological warfare programmes this century: the simple sabotage campaigns of the First World War; the major-state programmes of the middle years of the century; and the Soviet programme following the agreement of the BTWC, where the use of genetic engineering was significant. By the 1990s, therefore, analysts considered the threat from chemical and biological

Table 8.7   The CBW spectrum*

Chemicals
Classical CW:
  Mustard gas
  Nerve gas

Emerging CW:
  Toxic industrial chemicals
  Toxic pharmaceutical chemicals
  Toxic agricultural chemicals

Bioregulators:
  Peptides

Toxins:
  Saxitoxin
  Mycotoxin
  Ricin

Biological Organisms:
  Genetically manipulated BW
  Modified/tailored bacteria, viruses

Traditional BW:
  Bacteria
  Viruses
  Rickettsia

* From Office of Technology Assessment, *Biotechnology in a Global Economy* (see note 26).

Table 8.8   Illustrative list of potential BW agents*

Bacteria, Rickettsia, Chlamydia, Fungi, Viruses:
  Yersinia pestis, Bacillus anthracis, Pseudomonas mallei, Pseudomonas pseudomallei, Francisella tularensis, Brucella melitensis, Vibrio cholerae, Legionella pneumophilia... [30 in total]

Toxins of microorganisms:
  Botulinum toxins, enterotoxin A *Staphylococcus aureus*, alpha-toxin *Staphylococcus aureus*, neurotoxin *Shigella dysenteriae*

Toxins of animal origin:
  Tetrodotoxin, conotoxins, batrachotoxin

Toxins of plants and seaweed toxins:
  Abrin, ricin, saxitoxin;

Toxins of snakes and spiders:
  Taipoxin, textilotoxin... [11 in total]

Neuropeptides:
  Endothelin...

* From Geissler, 'A New Generation of Biological Weapons' (see note 27).

weapons to come from a wide spectrum of possibilities.[31] Table 8.7 sets out the categories of the spectrum. The biological agents are specified in more detail in, for example, an official Russian paper[32] prepared for the VEREX process (Table 8.8). This was a process in which an assessment was made of the scientific possibilities of verifying the BTWC.

This brief resumé of the history of biological warfare strongly suggests that if there are offensive military programmes today and in the future they will almost certainly use the capabilities made available by the ongoing revolution in biology and medicine. What then are the future possibilities?

Biological weapons in the near future

Mark Wheelis has proposed a three-point typology of possible biological warfare[33] involving the nature of the aggressor, the scale of release of agent and the identity of the target (Table 8.9). Within each dimension of this typology he then describes three possibilities. By combining the nature of the aggressor with the scale of release it is therefore possible to produce a nine-cell matrix of possible kinds of warfare (Table 8.10). It is obvious that biological weapons have a wide range of potential uses from small-scale criminal acts through to use as weapons of mass destruction.

Our concern here is primarily with possible military attacks on people. In the view of the US military there are four general categories of Concepts of Use (COU) which need to be considered: superpower *vs* superpower; state *vs* state; state *vs* factional element or *vice versa*; and

---

Table 8.9   Dimensions of biological warfare*

1. *Nature of the aggressor*
   a. Nations
   b. Subnational groups
   c. Individuals

2. *Scale of release*
   a. Point source release
   b. Medium-scale release
   c. Large-scale release

3. *Target*
   a. Human
   b. Plants
   c. Animals

---

* From Preston, 'Annals of Warfare' (see note 7).

terrorist use. These possibilities are described in more detail in Table 8.11. We are clearly no longer in a situation in which two massive superpowers are preparing for the possibility of all-out world war.

Table 8.10   Types of biological warfare*

Scale of release	Nature of aggressor		
	Individual	*Subnational group*	*State*
Point source	e.g. Criminal act	e.g. Assassination	e.g. Assassination
Medium scale tactical	e.g. Criminal	e.g. Terrorist	e.g. Military
Large scale strategic	Not possible	e.g. National liberation (army) use	e.g. Military

* From R. Preston, 'Annals of Warfare' (see note 7).

Table 8.11   Military concepts of use of biological weapons*

Superpower vs Superpower
'During periods of the cold war . . . the offensive programs of the two countries were orientiated principally towards use on a scale commensurate with this perceived threat. Programs on this scale would be expected to be highly sophisticated, difficult to disguise completely . . . and to require extensive facilities. . . . In addition to including smaller-scale weapons and simple delivery systems, a superpower BW program could include munitions delivery systems that are highly efficient, sophisticated, and provide large area coverage capability'.

State vs State
'In a conflict between two less technologically advanced countries . . . BW weapons might be desired and used by one country against another. In this COU, the quantities of agents needed for a limited number of weapons are likely to be far less than in a superpower program, and the types of delivery and dissemination equipment could be far less sophisticated. . . . The BW weapons are likely to be less efficient, more modest in sophistication and provide limited area coverage'.

State vs Factional Element or vice-versa
'In this COU, e.g., Iraq vs the Kurds, the targets are more limited, the quantities of agent needed are likely to be far less and the types of delivery and dissemination equipment could approach the primitive, yet still accomplish the goal . . . '

Terrorist Use
Terrorist use of BW agents could be as simple as a knowledgeable individual with a grudge, or as complex as State-sponsored terrorism. The quantities of agent could be small . . . production and purification methods extremely simple, and dissemination means simple to complex . . . '

* From Dando, 'New Developments in Biotechnology' (see note 24).

However, the world system remains in a transitional stage in which there must be a strong presumption of further state *vs* state and state *vs* factional element warfare. In such state *vs* state warfare: '... personnel of strategic facilities, eg ports, airbases, command posts, etc, could be targets during a tactical situation. Tactical applications against selected groups of unprotected troops by an unexpected attack can be envisaged...'[34]

It is not too difficult, therefore, to see why *Jane's Defence Weekly* argued that:

> much of the basis for US national security strategy and military planning today centres on the premise that the next time US troops deploy to a contingency in the Persian Gulf they must deal with the threat of WMD, and particularly chemical and biological weapons.[35]

The classical agents such as anthrax and botulinal toxin would obviously be a severe threat, but what else is of concern to the United States today?

We can gain an insight into the answer to that question from the technical annex to the US Secretary of State's report, *Proliferation: Threat and Response*, published in late 1997.[36] The potential novel agents said to be of concern are set out in Table 8.12. As the report makes clear, the extreme lethality of biological agents has long been recognized and the possibility of modifying the agents by means of the new genetic engineering techniques was envisaged as soon as the techniques were developed. However, lethality is only one of the requirements for an effective agent:

> Numerous characteristics need to be controlled for a highly effective biological warfare agent. Historically, the accentuation of one characteristic often resulted in the attenuation of one or more other characteristics, possibly even rendering the modified agent ineffective as a weapon...

Now, the report states: 'Advances in biotechnology, genetic engineering, and related scientific fields provide increasing potential to control more of these factors, possibly leading to the ability to use biological warfare agents as tactical battlefield weapons.' So, at the same time as the likely military operations appear to require agents tailored for specific, smaller-scale use rather than the overwhelming large-scale use envisaged during the superpowers' Cold War, advances in technology have provided the means to make specific modifications to agents. In

Table 8.12   Novel agents that could be produced by genetic engineering*

- Benign microorganisms, genetically altered to produce a toxin, venom, or bioregulator.
- Microorganisms resistant to antibiotics, standard vaccines, and therapeutics.
- Microorganisms with enhanced aerosol and environmental stability.
- Immunologically-altered microorganisms able to defeat standard identification, detection, and diagnostic methods.
- Combinations of the above four types with improved delivery systems.

* From Pearson, 'The CBW Spectrum', (see note 31).

summary, the report concludes, in regard to the possibilities listed in Table 8.12:

> It is noteworthy that each of these techniques seeks to capitalise on the extreme lethality, virulence, or infectivity of biological warfare agents and exploit this potential by developing methods to deliver more efficiently and to control these agents on the battlefield.

Thus post-Cold War, *fourth-generation*, offensive biological warfare programmes, if developed, appear likely to involve such specific *tailoring of classical agents*. In that sense, the agent for the US civil defence exercise – the smallpox-Marburg virus – does not seem to be a realistic current possibility. But military offence and defence interactions will not stop where they are today.

Twenty-first century biological weapons

Since the 1991 Gulf War, when there was considerable concern about the unpreparedness of troops, even from advanced industrial countries, to deal with possible use of biological weapons, there has clearly been considerable investment in detection, identification and force protection measures, both in the United States[37] and among its allies.[38] There is also a growing effort to build on current knowledge of how to deal with diseases caused by the classical agents,[39] even going so far as seeking generic means of medical protection against pathogens.[40]

The result could well be an action/reaction process in which the evolving threat is countered by an evolving defence. As it is described in the technical annex to *Proliferation: Threat and Response*: 'The current level of sophistication for many biological agents is low but there is enormous potential – based on advances in modern biology, fermentation, and drug delivery technology – for making more sophisticated weapons.'[41] But: 'a vigorous and productive defensive program is possible and will do much to mitigate the risk to the United States and its allies.' While the classical agents pose the greatest current threat and, perhaps in modified forms, near-future threat, the report suggests that '[t]he question of what disease-causing organisms might supplant classic biological warfare agents is critical to understanding future biological warfare threats'.

Though it does not provide any indication of what those future threats might be, the report identifies a series of technological trends which, it is suggested, could influence them. These trends are described in the four points listed in Table 8.13. The first point clearly refers to the employment of vectors such as the modified vaccinia virus used to carry elements of other organisms that was discussed previously.[42] The second point refers to the continuing development of our understanding of the mechanisms of pathogenesis.[43] The third point is different in that it deals not with other organisms that may be of concern but with human bodily defence mechanisms against disease. The potential for a long-term action/reaction process in offence and defence is clearly inherent in the final point, in the contention that vaccine development may be improved 'to the point where classic biological warfare agents will offer less utility as a means of causing casualties'.

What kinds of new weaponry might be produced by this process – say in a *fifth-generation* offensive biological weapons programme[44] by the second or third decade of the twenty-first century? One possibility is related to the development of new incapacitant (so-called non-lethal) weapons.[45] These are agents which in expected concentrations would cause few

Table 8.13   Significant trends related to future biological weapons possibilities*

- Genetically engineered vectors in the form of modified infectious organisms will be increasingly employed as tools in medicine and the techniques will become more widely available.
- Strides will be made in understanding of infectious disease mechanisms and in the microbial genetics that are responsible for disease processes.
- An increased understanding of human immune system function and disease mechanisms will shed light on the circumstances that cause individual susceptibility to infectious disease.
- vaccines and antidotes will be improved over the long term, perhaps to the point where classical biological warfare agents will offer less utility as a means of causing casualties.

---

*From Pearson: 'The CBW Spectrum' (see note 31).

deaths but would render those affected temporarily incapable of carrying out their duties. In the run-up to the Third Review Conference of the BTWC in 1991 the Canadian Government produced a study entitled *Novel Toxins and Bioregulators: the Emerging Scientific and Technological Issues Relating to Verification and the Biological and Toxin Weapons Convention.*[46] It drew attention to the problems that could arise should increasing knowledge of the functions of bioregulatory peptides (short strings of amino acids) in the human body be misused to create new agents causing incapacitation. Such misuse of bioregulators is prohibited by the general purpose criterion of both the BTWC and the Chemical Weapons Convention. The whole question of the possible development and operational deployment of non-lethal weapons raises a series of complex questions, and warnings have been given that they may in fact be harbingers of a new form of technologically-driven arms race rather than a means of conducting a more benign mode of armed conflict.[47]

This concern is reinforced by the view expressed in the Canadian document that while the evolutionary competition between organisms possessing lethal toxins and their natural target organisms means it is unlikely that toxicity of lethal toxins can be enhanced, however the functions of bioregulators, which are involved in modulating cellular activities within an organism may be capable of enhancement. The report states: 'The significance of this is that, while it is unlikely that research may lead to more toxic lethal agents, it may be possible to make more effective incapacitating agents.'[48]

The same point is made quite clearly in the US contribution to the background paper on new scientific and technological developments prepared for the Fourth Review Conference of the BTWC in 1996.[49] In a section devoted to ongoing developments with the most potential for misuse over the next decade, the US contribution deals specifically with bioregulatory peptides. It states:

Peptides are precursors of proteins made up of amino acids. . . . They are active at very low concentrations (one part per billion or trillion) which makes their detection very difficult. *They can be successfully modified as agonists* (more active products) *or antagonists* (having a contrary activity) . . . [emphasis added]

The section continues:

Their range of activity covers the entire living system, from mental processes (e.g. endorphins) to many aspects of health such as control of mood, consciousness, temperature control, sleep or emotions, exerting regulatory effects on the body. Even a small imbalance in these natural substances could have serious consequences, inducing fear, fatigue, depression or incapacitation. These substances would be extremely difficult to detect but could cause serious consequences or even death if used improperly.

There thus appear to be many possible means of misuse that could be designed in the future.[50]

It is presumably partly in regard to such bioregulators and their modification that the Final Document of the Fourth Review Conference stated, in respect to the scope of the BTWC as set out in Article I:

> The Conference also reaffirms that the Convention unequivocally covers all microbial *or other biological agents* or toxins, naturally or artificially created or altered, *as well as their components*, whatever their origin or method of production, of types and in quantities that have no justification for prophylactic, protective or other peaceful purposes. [emphasis added][51]

Obviously there could be difficulties in using such bioregulatory agents in an aerosol, but there may be means of improving their environmental stability,[52] and there have been suggestions in the literature that micro-organisms could be modified in order to manufacture such bioregulatory agents once inside a victim.[53] In other words, a benign micro-organism could be used as a vector (Table 8.13, first point; Table 8.12, first point). While it remains difficult to pin down the exact functions of many known neuropeptides, it seems very likely that our knowledge of how to specifically modify their functions will continue to develop rapidly.[54] Moreover, there is evidence of continuing military interest in new non-lethal incapacitants.[55]

Clearly, another possibility that will arise in the minds of weapon systems designers is to attack the human immune system – the body's own defences (Table 8.13, third point). This is a very complex system which has evolved to keep pathogens at bay. It has two subdivisions, one non-specific and innate, the other specific and adaptive and concerned with *acquired immunity*.[56] This second subdivision: 'produces a specific response to each infectious agent, and the effector mechanisms generated normally eradicate the offending material. Furthermore the adaptive immune system remembers the particular infectious agent and can prevent it causing disease later'. This second specific part of the system also has two main components. Its response:

takes two forms, *humoral* and *cell-mediated*, which usually develop in parallel. . . . Humoral immunity depends on the appearance in the blood of antibodies produced by plasma cells. . . . Cell-mediated immunity depends mainly on the development of T cells that are specifically responsive to the inducing agent . . .

The cross-links between humoral and cell-mediated immunity are complex but depend, in part, on the activity of various cytokines (biologically active peptides and proteins that act near their site of release). The plasma cells that secrete antibodies into the blood are called B cells but, 'Many antigens do not stimulate antibody production without the help of T lymphocytes. These antigens first bind to the B cell, which must then be exposed to T cell-derived lymphokines [a form of cytokine], i.e. helper factors, before antibody can be produced.' During evolution pathogenic micro-organisms have developed ways of subverting the immune system. One recent survey noted that: '[m]ore than 50 different virus genes have been identified as immune modulators; this collection is certainly incomplete.' The weapons system designer would therefore have many leads to follow in developing ways to attack the system.

This can hardly be regarded as idle speculation about new forms of attack because, while it was not clear at that time, one of the agents weaponized in the US offensive biological warfare programme is now known to operate through a specific disruption of the human immune system. Staphylococcal enterotoxin B (SEB) is secreted as one of the exotoxins of *Staphylococcus aureus*.

Because these exotoxins are extremely potent activators of T cells, they are commonly referred to as bacterial superantigens. These superantigens stimulate the production and secretion of various cytokines from immune system cells. Released cytokines are thought to mediate most of the toxic effects of SEB.[57]

When used as a biological weapon by inhalation exposure very small amounts of SEB would cause enough over-production of cytokines to render exposed people ill within a few hours. Incapacitation would last from several days to weeks and involve fever, headache etc. of a severe nature. However, it could be that much more effective means of attack will be possible in the future since studies of the role of superantigens are 'in their infancy' at the present time.[58]

Conclusion

The illustrations just given of the ways in which our increasing knowledge of molecular medicine might allow directed specific attacks on human beings are only some of the many possibilities. As the 48th General Assembly of the World Medical Association pointed out in its 1996 statement, 'Weapons and their relation to life and health':

> The potential for scientific and medical knowledge to contribute to the development of new weapons systems, targeted against specific individuals, specific populations or against body systems, is considerable. This could include the development of weapons designed to target anatomical or physiological systems ... [59]

Thus, although traditional, proven, classical agents will continue to present the greatest danger for some time to come, the 'extreme scenario' examined at the start of this paper will not be extreme for long if offensive military biological weapons programmes are allowed to continue under a weak BTWC. Our task is to find effective means of stopping all such programmes and to build confidence in compliance with the Convention.

Notes

1   J. Miller and W. J. Broad, 'Secret Exercise Finds US Can't Cope with a Biological Terror Attack', *International Herald Tribune*, 27 April 1998, p. 3.
2   M. Meselson, and J. P. Perry Robinson, 'Outline for an Integrated Approach to the Problem of Biological Weapons', Paper presented to Pugwash Meeting No. 212, Geneva, 2–3 December 1995.
3   J. Jelama, 'Military Implications of Biotechnology', in M. Fransman et al. (eds), *The Biotechnology Revolution* (Oxford: Blackwell, 1995) pp. 284–97.
4   M. R. Dando, *Biological Warfare in the 21st Century* (London: Brassey's, 1994).
5   L. Collier, L. and J. Oxford, *Human Virology* (Oxford: Oxford University Press, 1993).
6   United Kingdom, 'New Scientific and Technological Developments Relevant to the Biological and Toxin Weapons Convention', in *Background Paper on New Scientific and Technological Developments Relevant to the Convention on the Prohibition of the Development, Production and Stockpiling of Bacteriological (Biological) and Toxin Weapons and on their Destruction*. BWC/CONF.IV/4 (Geneva: United Nations, 1996) pp. 7–18.
7   R. Preston, 'Annals of Warfare: the Bioweaponeers', *New Yorker*, March 1998, pp. 52–65.

8   Ibid.
9   B. Starr, 'DARPA Begins Research to Counter Biological Pathogens', *Jane's Defence Weekly* (15 October 1997) p. 8.
10 H. Smith, 'The Mounting Interest in Bacterial and Viral Pathogenicity', *Annual Review of Microbiology*, 43 (1989) pp. 1–22.
11 A. J. Cann, *Principles of Molecular Virology* (London: Academic Press, 1993).
12 E. G. Stockwell, 'Infant Mortality', in K. E. Kiple (ed.), *The Cambridge History of Human Disease* (Cambridge: Cambridge University Press, 1993) pp. 224–9.
13 J. A. Poupard and L. A. Miller, 'History of Biological Warfare: Catapults to Capsomeres', *Annals of the New York Academy of Sciences*, 666 (1992) pp. 9–19.
14 M. Wheelis, 'Biological Warfare Before 1914: the Prescientific Era', in E. Geissler and J. E. van Courtland Moon (eds), *Biological and Toxin Weapons Research, Development and Use from the Middle Ages to 1945: a Critical Comparative Analysis* (Oxford: Oxford University Press, for SIPRI, 1998).
15 M. Wheelis, 'Biological Sabotage in the First World War', in ibid.
16 O. Lepick, 'French Activities Related to Biological Warfare: 1919–1945', in ibid.
17 S. H. Harris, *Factories of Death: Japanese Biological Warfare 1932–45 and the American Cover Up* (London: Routledge, 1994).
18 Scientific and Technical Advisory Section G. H. Q., AFPAC, *Report on Scientific Intelligence Survey in Japan (September and October 1945). Volume V: Biological Warfare*. Report No. BIOS/JAP/PR/746, British Intelligence Objectives Sub-Committee (London: HMSO, 1945).
19 G. B. Carter, 'Biological Warfare and Biological Defence in the United Kingdom 1940–1979', *Journal of the Royal United Services Institute* (December 1992) pp. 67–74.
20 C. S. Cox, *The Aerobiological Pathway of Microorganisms* (Chichester: John Wiley, 1987).
21 P. H. Gregory, *The Microbiology of the Atmosphere*, 2nd edn (London: Leonard Hill, 1973).
22 Joint Technical Warfare Committee, *Potentialities of Weapons of War During the Next Ten Years* (TWC (45) 42) 12 November 1945.
23 US Army, *US Army Activity in the US Biological Warfare Programs, vols I and II.* (Washington DC: Department of the Army, 24 February 1977).
24 M. R. Dando, 'New Developments in Biotechnology and their Impact on Biological Warfare', in O. Thränert (ed.), *Enhancing the Biological Weapons Convention* (Bonn: Dietz, 1996) pp. 21–56.
25 US Army (1977), *US Army Activity*, op. cit.
26 Office of Technology Assessment, *Biotechnology in a Global Economy* OTA-BA-494. (Washington DC: US Congress, 1991).
27 E. Geissler, 'A New Generation of Biological Weapons', in E. Geissler (ed.), *Biological and Toxin Weapons Today* (Oxford: Oxford University Press for SIPRI, 1986) pp 21–35.
28 R. Preston, 'Annals of Warfare', op. cit.
29 M. R. Dando, *Biological Warfare*, op. cit.
30 R. Preston, 'Annals of Warfare', op. cit.
31 G. S. Pearson, 'The CBW Spectrum', *The ASA Newsletter*, 90 (1) (1990) pp. 1; 7–8.
32 Russian Federation, *Illustrative List of Potential BW Agents* BWC/CONF.III/VEREX/WP.23 (Geneva: United Nations, 1992).

33 M. Wheelis, 'Addressing the Full Range of Biological Warfare in a BWC Compliance Protocol', Paper presented at Pugwash Meeting No. 229, *Strengthening the Biological Weapons Convention*, Geneva, 20–21 September 1997.
34 R. O. Spetzel et al., *Biological Weapons: Technical Report*, DNA-MIPR-90–715 (Fort Detrick, Md.: US Army Medical Research Institute of Infectious Diseases, 1994).
35 B. Starr, 'Countering Weapons of Mass Destruction', *Jane's Defence Weekly* (12 November 1997) pp. 39–40.
36 W. Cohen, *Proliferation: Threat and Response* (Washington DC: Department of Defense (Text from WorldWideWebsite http://www.defenselink.mil/pubs/prolif97/index.html).
37 W. L. Busbee, 'Chemical and Biological Threats and Responses: a U.S. Perspective', Paper presented at the 6th International Symposium on Protection Against Chemical and Biological Warfare Agents, 10–15 May 1998, Stockholm. FOA-R-98-00749-862-SE.
38 B. Roberts and G. S. Pearson, 'Bursting the Biological Bubble: How Prepared are We for Biowar?' *Jane's International Defence Review*, 4 (1998) pp. 21–4.
39 D. Franz et al., 'Clinical Recognition and Management of Patients Exposed to Biological Warfare Agents', *Journal of the American Medical Association*, 278 (5) (1997) pp. 399–411.
40 S. B. Jones, 'Unconventional Pathogen Countermeasures', Paper presented at the 6th International Symposium on Protection Against Chemical and Biological Warfare Agents, 10–15 May 1998, Stockholm. FOA-R-98-00749-862-SE.
41 W. Cohen, *Proliferation*, op. cit.
42 L. Collier and J. Oxford, *Human Virology*, op. cit.
43 H. Smith, 'The Mounting Interest', op. cit.
44 M. R. Dando, 'Advances in Biotechnology: Their Relevance to the Task of Strengthening the Biological and Toxin Weapons Convention', Paper presented to a NATO Advanced Studies Institute on New Scientific and Technological Aspects of Verification of the Biological and Toxin Weapons Convention (BTWC), 11–18 June 1997, Budapest.
45 M. R. Dando, *A New Form of Warfare: the Rise of Non-Lethal Weapons* (London: Brassey's, 1996).
46 Canada, *Novel Toxins and Bioregulators: the Emerging Scientific and Technological Issues Relating to Verification and the Biological and Toxin Weapons Convention* (Ottawa, September 1991).
47 R. Coupland, '"Non-lethal" Weapons: Precipitating a New Arms Race', *British Medical Journal*, Editorial (12 July 1997) p. 72.
48 Canada, *Novel Toxins*, op. cit.
49 United States, *Background Paper on New Scientific and Technological Developments Relevant to the Convention on the Prohibition of the Development, Production and Stockpiling of Bacteriological (Biological) and Toxin Weapons and on their Destruction* BWC/CONF.IV/4 (Geneva: United Nations, 1996) pp. 18–26.
50 M. R. Dando (1994), op. cit.; M. R. Dando, 'New Developments in Biotechnology', op. cit.
51 United Nations, *Final Document: Fourth Review Conference of the Parties to the Convention on the Prohibition of the Development, Production and Stockpiling of Bacteriological (Biological) and Toxin Weapons and on their Destruction.* BWC/CONF.IV/9 (Geneva: United Nations, 1996).

52 Canada, *Novel Toxins*, op. cit.
53 B. Starr, 'Bioagents Could Target Ethnic Groups, Says CIA', *Jane's Defence Weekly* (25 June 1997) p. 6.
54 C. Betancur et al., 'Nonpeptide Antagonists of Neuropeptide Receptors: Tools for Research and Therapy', *TiPS*, 18 (1997) pp. 372–86; N. Bedor and P. Buchwald, 'All in the Mind', *Chemistry in Britain* (January 1998) pp. 36–9.
55 C. Beal, 'Briefing: Non-lethal Weapons', *Jane's Defence Weekly* (24 June 1998) pp. 23–5.
56 J. Stewart and D. M. Weir, 'Innate and Acquired Immunity', in D. Greenwood et al. (eds), *Medical Microbiology*, 15th edn (Edinburgh: Churchill Livingstone, 1997) pp. 119–45.
57 D. Franz et al., op. cit.
58 A. Weiss and L. J. Miller, 'Halting the March of the Immune Defenses', editorial introduction to articles on 'Turning the Immune System Off', *Science*, 280 (10 April 1998) p. 179.
59 World Medical Assembly, *Statement: Weapons and their Relation to Life and Health*. 48th WMA General Assembly, 20–26 October 1996, Somerset West, South Africa.

9

Non-Medical Aspects of Emerging and Re-emerging Infectious Diseases: Maximum Protection with Minimal Disruption

David Heymann

The global community

The processes of globalization and technological innovation have resulted in the mixing of human populations to a level unprecedented in human history. Over 52 million persons travel by air from industrialized to developing countries each year. In addition, increased numbers of people from developing countries are travelling to industrialized countries for reasons of commerce, education and tourism. International migration has been for both voluntary and involuntary reasons, as conditions of turmoil and civil strife have resulted in an estimated 26 million refugees, in 1996, residing in countries in which they had not previously lived. This constant mixing of human populations has made the world a true global community.

The globalization of human populations has repercussions on other ecological systems, particularly those of the microbial world. Disease-causing microbes often accompany travellers, and as a result infectious diseases, some of which are resistant to treatment, are spreading throughout the world. At the dawn of the twenty-first century, humans, like mosquitoes, have become efficient vectors of disease, transferring disease-causing microbes from one continent to another in a matter of hours. During 1996, for example, yellow fever was imported in tourists from Latin America to North America and Europe; in 1992 an antibiotic-resistant microbe (*Streptococcus pneumoniae*) which causes common adult pneumonia was transferred by travellers from a European country to the Americas, Africa and Asia. In 1994, Ebola infection was imported to Europe from West Africa, and in 1997 Ebola infection travelled from western to southern Africa. Increases in trade and travel have facilitated the spread of endemic as well as new unusual emerging infectious diseases to new virgin territories.

International legislation to ensure maximum protection with minimal disruption

The transfer of disease from one country to another with travel is not new. In 1377 the first recorded quarantine legislation was written in the city of Venice, to protect the city from plague-carrying rats on ships from foreign ports. Similar legislation in Europe, and later the Americas and other regions, led to the first international sanitary conference in 1851. This conference was driven by concerns regarding the spread of infectious disease, as well as national concerns regarding the disruption of international trade by quarantine restrictions. This conference laid down the still valid principle for protection against the international spread of infectious diseases: maximum protection with minimum restriction. Although uniform quarantine measures were determined at that time, a full century elapsed before the International Sanitary Rules were adopted by the World Health Organization (WHO) in 1951. These were amended in 1969 to become the existing International Health Regulations (IHR).

The IHR provide a universal code of practice to standardize the procedures to be followed by all countries in controlling infectious diseases of international importance and their potential for international spread. They specify what should be done by whom and for what purpose. These include the development of strong national disease detection systems, as well as specific measures of disease prevention and control including vaccinations, disinfection, and de-ratting. Currently, the IHR require the reporting of just three infectious diseases – cholera, plague and yellow fever – and they delineate the specific measures that nations are allowed to take in relation to outbreaks of these diseases.

Despite IHR guidelines for action, past misapplication of the Regulations in response to disease notification by states has resulted in distortions of international travel and trade, and consequent huge economic losses to the states involved. In 1991, the present pandemic of cholera reached Latin America and was identified in Peru. As required by the IHR, Peru immediately notified WHO of this outbreak. During that year alone, cholera infected over 300 000 people, resulting in 3000 deaths in Peru. In addition to this enormous public health impact, the epidemic also led to severe trade (due to concerns about food safety) and tourism losses as neighbouring nations and trading partners imposed measures in excess of those permitted by the International Health Regulations. Estimated losses to the Peruvian economy are as high as 770 million US dollars. The Peruvian example clearly illustrates the misapplication of the IHR, in that disease notification for the purposes of maximum protection was not accompanied by measures allowing only the minimum restriction of international trade.

In 1994 an outbreak of plague occurred in India with approximately 1000 presumptive cases. The appearance of pneumonic plague resulted in thousands of Indians fleeing from the outbreak area, risking spread of the disease to new areas. Plague did not spread but the outbreak led to tremendous economic disruption and concern worldwide, compounded by the misinterpretation and misapplication of the IHR. Nations closed airports to aeroplanes arriving from India, exports of foodstuffs were blocked, and in some countries Indian guest workers were forced to return to India even though they had not been there for several years. It is estimated that the nation sustained economic losses as high as 1700 million US dollars. Again, as a result of the misapplication of the IHR, the country suffered negative consequences of reporting an IHR-mandated disease.

A further problem identified in the existing IHR is that many infectious diseases, including those which are new or emerging, are not covered despite their great potential for international spread. In 1995 an outbreak of Ebola haemorrhagic fever occurred in Zaire in which 316 cases and 245 deaths occurred. The immediate reaction of the national government was to close the road leading from Kinshasa (the capital city) to the outbreak site 500 kilometres away, in order to contain the epidemic. A 24-hour police barrier was established on the road, but the airport near the outbreak site, and the river passing through the site which eventually reaches the capital, were not part of the quarantine and indeed a case of Ebola did arrive in the capital city by air. Fortunately, strengthened disease surveillance in Kinshasa immediately detected the case and no local spread occurred. Had this person with Ebola infection boarded an international flight in Kinshasa, the IHR could not have been applied to contain its spread. In fact, the international spread of Ebola has already occurred, with the 1997 case of a patient with Ebola infection who travelled from western Africa and subsequently transmitted the infection to a hospital nurse in southern Africa. In such instances, when outbreaks of infectious diseases not covered by the IHR occur there is great uncertainty nationally and internationally as to what measures should be taken.

In 1993 an outbreak of a disease characterized by fever, muscle aches and intestinal complaints followed by the abrupt onset of shortness of breath and rapid progression to death was first identified in the southwestern United States. Cases were soon identified in other southwestern states and the cause was found to be a newly identified virus in the Hantavirus family. The epidemic was shown to be associated with a mouse now known to be its reservoir. Although there was great national alarm as a result of this outbreak and concern about the possibility of cross-border transmission, the limited scope of the existing Regulations meant that no international legal guideline existed pertaining to which measures were appropriate to contain the international spread of the organism.

Because of the problematic application and limited disease coverage of the IHR, WHO has undertaken a revision and updating of the IHR to make them more applicable to infection control in future. The revised Regulations will replace reporting of specific diseases with the reporting of disease syndromes, for example, current legislation requiring the reporting of cholera will be replaced with the reporting of syndromes of epidemic diarrhoeal disease with high mortality. As a result, the IHR will have a broader scope to include all infectious diseases of international importance, and will clearly indicate what measures are appropriate internationally, as well as those which are inappropriate. The revised IHR will aim to control disease at the site of the outbreak rather than through the imposition of barriers at borders, which in the globalized environment are of negligible public health significance and create a false sense of security that infectious disease will not enter.

The underlying problem

The International Health Regulations alone cannot control the spread of infectious diseases. Prevention, and early detection and containment of the emergence and re-emergence of infectious diseases are also required. The infrastructure for infectious disease prevention, surveillance and control has weakened during the past twenty years and in some cases become ineffective. This has been compounded by concurrent changes in population, the environment and human behaviour.

Weakening of the public health infrastructure for infectious disease control can be seen to a greater or lesser extent in most countries. It is clearly evidenced by failures such as the lack of mosquito control in Latin America and Asia and the consequent re-emergence of major epidemics of dengue, a mosquito-borne viral disease; the failure of vaccination programmes in eastern Europe which have contributed to the re-emergence of epidemic diphtheria and polio; and the neglect of yellow fever vaccination, facilitating yellow fever outbreaks in Latin America and sub-Saharan Africa.

At the same time, population increases and rapid urbanization have resulted in increased burdens on public health systems already struggling to cope, resulting in a breakdown of sanitation and water systems in large coastal cities in Latin America, Asia and Africa and leading to epidemics of infectious diseases, such as the cholera outbreak described previously. In 1950, there were only two urban areas in the world with populations greater than seven million, but by 1990 this number had risen to 23 with increasing populations in and around all major cities challenging the capacity of existing sanitary systems.

Man-made or natural changes in the environment and in patterns of human interaction in the global ecosystem have also contributed to the emergence and re-emergence of infectious diseases. Changes range from global warming and consequent extension of vector-borne diseases, to ecological changes including deforestation that increase contact between man and animals, resulting in an increased possibility for micro-organisms to breach the species barrier. These are changes that have occurred on almost every continent. They are exemplified by zoonotic diseases such as Lassa fever, which was first identified in West Africa 1969 and is now known to be transmitted to man from human food supplies contaminated with the urine of rats in search of food that their natural habitat can no longer provide. The desert zone in sub-Saharan Africa, in which epidemic meningitis traditionally occurs, has grown larger as drought spreads south, bringing with it epidemic meningitis to countries such as Uganda and Tanzania.

Alterations in human behaviour have also played a role in the emergence and re-emergence of infectious diseases, best exemplified by the increase in gonorrhoea and syphilis during the late 1970s, and the emergence and amplification of HIV worldwide. The development of anti-microbial resistance to usual antibiotic treatment is further eroding our capacity to control infectious diseases, partly occurring as a result of the indiscriminate use of antibiotics. Antibiotic resistance adversely affects the treatment of patients with common infectious diseases such as pneumonia, gonorrhoea, tuberculosis and dysentery.

International and national response

In an optimal international human environment, the eradication or elimination of infectious diseases would ensure maximum protection against infectious diseases while preventing human suffering and death, obviating the need for the International Health Regulations. However, despite the advances of medical technology, very few infectious diseases are candidates for eradication. Diseases which can be eradicated or eliminated must have no reservoir other than humans, and provide solid immunity after infection. At the same time, an affordable and effective intervention must be available.

There are diseases that have been successfully eradicated, and WHO has targeted a list of diseases whose incidence is declining and are candidates for eradication in the next few decades. The eradication of smallpox was achieved in 1977 and certified in 1980. Transmission of poliomyelitis has been interrupted in the Americas and the disease is expected to be eradicated from the world during the coming decade. During 1996, 2090 cases of polio were reported to WHO, a decrease from 32 251 cases reported in 1988. Reported cases of dracunculiasis have decreased from over 900 000 in 1989 to less than 200 000 in 1996 with the majority of cases in one endemic country. Leprosy and Chagas disease likewise continue their downward trends towards elimination.

In the absence of eradication and elimination, which applies to very few infectious diseases, other measures are required to ensure maximum protection. These include: rebuilding the weakened public health infrastructure and strengthening water and sanitary systems; minimizing the impact of natural and man-made changes of the environment; effectively communicating information about prevention of infectious diseases; and appropriately using antibiotics to slow the evolution of antimicrobial resistance. However, even if these measures are applied with total commitment, the resilient nature of the microbial world, able to adapt to the evolutionary pressures of a changing environment, dictates that infectious diseases will continue to emerge and re-emerge. The issue is not eradication, but rather the development of effective international health mechanisms to cope with infectious disease.

Thus, there are two means of ensuring maximum protection from infectious diseases with minimal disruption: applying the International Health Regulations, and strengthening public health infrastructure for better prevention, detection and control of infectious diseases where they occur. Both are important. The inherent weakness in the IHR is that they come into application only after infectious diseases have become a threat, and are then subject to interpretation by sovereign nations which themselves decide on whether and how they should be applied. If applied as intended in their revised form, they will remain an important tool for international response as countries undertake the process to rebuild public health infrastructure, and prevent or detect and stop infectious diseases where they occur. International and national solidarity in the application of the IHR and in rebuilding the networks able to prevent, detect and contain infectious diseases will minimize their impact on human health, travel and trade.

Suggested Reading

W. A. Ashford et al., 'Penicillinase-Producing *Neisseria gonorrhoeae*', *Lancet*, 2 (1976) pp. 657–8.

N. Aswapokee et al., 'Pattern of Antibiotic Use in Medical Wards of a University Hospital, Bangkok, Thailand', *Review of Infectious Diseases*, 12 (1990) pp. 136–41.

R. P. Bax, 'Antibiotic Resistance: a View from the Pharmaceutical Industry', *Clinical Infectious Diseases*, 24(Supp. 1) (1997) S151–S153.

Siméant S. Choléra, 'Viel Ennemi, Nouveau Visage', *World Health Statistics Quarterly*, 45(2/3) (1992) pp. 208–19.

'Ebola Haemorrhagic Fever', *Weekly Epidemiological Record*, 70(34) (1995) pp. 241–2.

'Ebola Haemorrhagic Fever: a Summary of the Outbreak in Gabon', *Weekly Epidemiological Record* 72.5 (1997) pp. 7–8.

Ebola Haemorrhagic Fever in Zaire, 1976: Report of an International Commission', *Bulletin of the World Health Organization*, 56(2) (1978) pp. 270–93.

Expanded Programme on Immunization (EPI), 'Update: Diptheria Epidemic in the Newly Independent States of the Former USSR, January 1995–March 1996', *Weekly Epidemiological Record*, 71(33) (1996) pp. 245–50.

F. Fenner et al., *Smallpox and its Eradication* (Geneva: WHO, 1988).

Goma Epidemiology Group, 'Public Health Impact of Rwandan Refugee Crisis: What Happened in Goma, Zaire, in July, 1994?' *Lancet*, 345 (1995) pp. 339–44.

The Gonococcal Antimicrobial Surveillance Programme (GASP), 'WHO Western Pacific Region, 1995', *Weekly Epidemiological Record*, 72(5) (1997) pp. 25–7.

D. L. Heymann and G. Rodier, 'Remerging Pathogens and Diseases out of Control', *Lancet*, 349 (Supp. 3) (1997) pp. 8–10.

S. D. Holmberg et al., 'Health and Economic Impact of Antimicrobial Resistance', *Review of Infectious Diseases*, 9 (1987) pp. 1065–78.

International Health Regulations, 3rd annotated edn (Geneva: World Health Organization, 1969).

J. Lederberg, R. E. Shope and S. C. Oaks (eds), *Emerging Infections: Microbial Threats to Health in the United States* (Washington, DC: Institute of Medicine/ National Academy Press, 1992).

S. C. Lester et al., 'The Carriage of *Escherichia coli* Resistant to Antimicrobial Agents by Healthy Children in Boston, in Caracas, Venezuela and Qin Pu, China', *New England Journal of Medicine*, 323 (1990) pp. 285–9.

S. B. Levy, *The Antibiotic Paradox: How Miracle Drugs are Destroying the Miracle* (New York: Plenum Press, 1992).

'Meningococcal Meningitis', *Weekly Epidemiological Record*, 70(15) (1995) pp. 105–7.

T. P. Monath, 'Lassa Fever: Review of Epidemiology and Epizootiology', *Bulletin of the World Health Organization*, 52 (1975) pp. 577–92.

R. Munoz et al., 'Intercontinental Spread of a Multiresistant Clone of Serotype 23F *Streptococcus pneumoniae*', *Journal of Infectious Diseases*, 164 (1991) pp. 302–6.

C. J. L. Murray and A. D. Lopez, *Global Health Statistics: a Compendium of Incidence, Prevalence and Mortality Estimates for Over 200 Conditions* (Cambridge, Mass.: Harvard School of Public Health on Behalf of WHO and the World Bank, 1996).

I. Phillips, 'β-Lactamase-Producing, Penicillin-Resistant Gonococcus', *Lancet*, 2 (1976) pp. 656–7.

'Poliomyelitis Outbreak', *Weekly Epidemiological Record*, 71(39) (1996) pp. 293–5.

S. E. Robertson et al., 'Yellow Fever: a Decade of Reemergence', *Journal of the American Medical Association*, 276(14) (1996) pp. 1157–62.

P. A. Sato et al., 'Review of AIDS and HIV Infection: Global Epidemiology and Statistics', *AIDS 1989*, 3 (Supp. 1) S301–S307.

S. Soares et al., 'Evidence for the Introduction of a Multiresistant Clone of 6B *Streptococcus pneumoniae* from Spain to Iceland in the late 1980s', *Journal of Infectious Diseases*, 168 (1993) pp. 158–63.

United Nations Centre for Human Settlements (HABITAT), *An Urbanizing World: Global Report on Human Settlements, 1996* (New York: United Nations, 1996).

'Update: Hantavirus Pulmonary Syndrome – United States, 1993', *Morbidity and Mortality Weekly Report*, 42(42) (1993) pp. 816–20.

J. N. Wasserheit, 'Effect of Changes in Human Ecology and Behavior on Patterns of Sexually Transmitted Diseases, including Human Immunodeficiency Virus Infection', *Proceedings of the National Academy of Sciences*, 91 (1994) pp. 2430–5.

'World Malaria Situation in 1993, Part 1', *Weekly Epidemiological Record*, 71(3) (1996) pp. 17–22.

10
Challenges to the World Health Organization

*Yves Beigbeder**

As part of a weakened United Nations system, the World Health Organization (WHO) is currently facing a serious credibility crisis, together with a financial crisis. This is all the more surprising since WHO has long been considered a prestigious and efficient organization, enjoying a respected renown for scientific and medical expertise and widely acclaimed for its victory over smallpox. Run by capable leaders, who avoided major political conflicts, WHO was regarded as the best managed UN specialized agency, with a solid financial backing assuring regular growth.

However, in recent years, the main donor governments have expressed concern about the Organization's management, leadership and effectiveness. Political and economic pressures in the countries which contribute most to the budget of WHO have caused a reappraisal of the role of the organization, together with financial cuts used as incentives for reform or as signs of dissatisfaction with programmes and/or management. A number of independent groups have assessed the strengths and weaknesses of WHO and proposed remedies.

At the same time, challenges to public health at the national and international levels are growing. In particular, new and re-emerging infectious diseases are threatening the health of populations in industrialized and developing countries. During the past two decades, at least 29 new infectious diseases have appeared, including the HIV virus, Ebola haemorrhagic fever and legionnaires' disease. Older diseases like tuberculosis, dengue fever and diphtheria that had gone into decline are returning with renewed vigour, a problem complicated by the growing phenomenon of antibiotic resistance. For WHO, key factors in the upsurge of disease have been the weakening of traditional public health activities around the world, especially surveillance, and the deteriorating condition of public health laboratories needed to identify emerging problems quickly. The potential of epidemics to spread has increased, due to the growing number of overcrowded cities with poor water and sanitation, migration and the flows of refugees, the deterioration or collapse of health systems in some countries, the increase in international travel, changes in global food trade and climate change.

Can WHO respond effectively and at reasonable cost to these old and new challenges? Is WHO fulfilling its constitutional mandate as the 'directing and co-ordinating authority on international health work'? Is WHO giving value for money? Could other less costly and more effective organizations give similar or better services? Rivals to WHO have already assumed some of its functions.

New and re-emerging infectious diseases

In its *World Health Report* 1996, WHO stated that infectious diseases are the world's leading cause of death, killing at least 17 million people a year, most of them young children. Up to half the six billion people on earth are at risk of many endemic diseases. Among the new diseases:

- the AIDS virus, predominantly transmitted sexually, has already infected up to 24 million adults, of whom at least four million have died. By the end of the century, WHO estimates that between 30 and 40 million men, women and children will have been infected with HIV;
- viral hepatitis is rapidly emerging as another global health issue. At least 350 million people are chronic carriers of the hepatitis B virus and another 100 million are chronic carriers of the hepatitis C virus. Up to a quarter of them will die of related liver disease. The hepatitis E virus is a major cause of acute hepatitis;
- new deadly haemorrhagic fevers have appeared in several continents. Among them, Ebola was first identified in Zaire and Sudan in 1976 and emerged again in Zaire in 1995: it was fatal in about 80 per cent of cases.

Among the main re-emerging diseases:

- malaria remains a major global target for action, with an annual incidence of between 300 and 500 million clinical cases, African countries south of the Sahara accounting for more than 90 per cent of cases;

- tuberculosis kills approximately three million people annually. Case notifications increased by 28 per cent during the 1990–3 period compared to 1984–6;
- cholera, dengue, diphtheria, bubonic plague and diarrhoeas are also cited by WHO. Seven out of every ten deaths in developing countries are due to just five causes: pneumonia, diarrhoea, malaria, measles and malnutrition.

WHO has initiated campaigns for the eradication of specific diseases, with diverse measures of success and failure. As a credible alternative to a difficult or impossible eradication, WHO has aimed at the elimination of leprosy 'as a public health problem'. Other campaigns are, more modestly, systematic efforts to control diseases.

WHO's past and present eradication campaigns

The failure of malaria eradication

WHO launched its first major eradication campaign in 1955, against malaria. Between 1959 and 1966, financial obligations for malaria eradication accounted for 10.8 per cent of WHO's regular budget and 27.2 per cent of all funds placed at the Organization's disposal. An estimated $1400 million was spent on the programme between 1957 and 1967, for which WHO provided technical leadership. International health consultants from Geneva and the Regional Offices advised national Health Ministries on the practicability and implementation of the programme. By 1965, there were 381 WHO malaria advisory staff involved in country or regional projects.[1] It was a 'vertical' programme carried out by international specialists and specialized units in Health Ministries. Eradication failed in front of an accumulation of technical, operational, financial and political problems, and in particular, the resistance of malaria vectors to insecticides. In 1969, the World Health Assembly revised the strategy of malaria eradication and stressed the need for the involvement of national health services in the programme. It recommended that although eradication should remain the ultimate goal, in countries where eradication was not possible, malaria control operations could provide a transitional stage.

WHO's current and more limited role is one of surveillance of the disease, advice to Health Ministries and encouragement to research for an effective vaccine. A 1992 Conference approved a global malaria strategy with the following basic technical elements: provision of early diagnosis and prompt treatment for the disease; planning and implementation of selective and sustainable preventive measures, including vector control; early detection for the prevention or containment of epidemics; and strengthening of local research capacities to promote regular reassessment of countries' malaria situations, in particular the ecological, social and economic determinants of the disease.

Donor countries helped finance the WHO malaria control programme in the amount of $3.5 million for 1993–4.

Smallpox eradication: the successful crusade

WHO's success in eradicating smallpox is well known. In 1966 the World Health Assembly launched the programme; and in 1979 a Global Commission certified the worldwide eradication of smallpox, the last known natural case having occurred in 1977. As for the Malaria Eradication Programme, the Smallpox Eradication Programme was directed centrally from WHO headquarters. 687 international staff from 73 countries worked on the programme, assisted by volunteers, plus approximately 150 000 staff of Health Ministries. The costs of the campaign, at national and international levels, amounted to approximately $313 million, while savings to countries from now unnecessary vaccination and medical care for smallpox patients were estimated at $1 billion a year.[2]

The eradication of poliomyelitis

In 1988, the World Health Assembly established a target to eradicate poliomyelitis worldwide by the year 2000. The countries undertaking polio eradication are supported by a coalition of partners which includes WHO and UNICEF, the US Centers for Disease Control and Prevention (CDC), and Rotary International. Most of the costs of polio eradication are borne by the countries themselves, with external assistance from industrialized countries and NGOs.

For 1995, global immunization coverage, which consists of three doses of Oral Polio Vaccine to all children under five years of age, was estimated by WHO at 83 per cent. The reported incidence of polio cases fell to 6179 in 1995. This represented a 28 per cent decline from 1994 and an 82 per cent decline from the 31 251 cases reported in 1988 when the eradication target was set. A total of 150 countries reported zero cases and seven countries failed to report. Because epidemiological surveillance is incomplete in many polio-endemic countries, WHO estimates that approximately 80 000 cases of paralytic polio occurred in 1995.

WHO provides the global technical leadership to this programme with a small staff at its headquarters in Geneva. UNICEF advocates globally for the programme and plays a key role in social mobilization. UNICEF is also a major provider of vaccines and immunization equipment and provides operational support in countries. CDC provides technical laboratory and programmatic assistance, as well as funds. Rotary's PolioPlus programme has collected and allocated $223 million in grants for immunization and eradication efforts in 111 countries, and has granted $5.3 million to the WHO programme. WHO estimates that the total amount of external resources still required to achieve and certify global polio eradication exceeds $500 million. Together with WHO and UNICEF, Rotary is leading international advocacy efforts to expand the partnership of organizations and governments supporting the polio initiative – in other words, to obtain the necessary additional voluntary funding.[3]

The planned eradication of dracunculiasis

Dracunculiasis (Guinea worm disease) has also been targeted by WHO for eradication, to be completed by the end of the 1990s. This parasitic disease is prevalent in 18 countries. In 1994 there were approximately 100 000 cases reported worldwide. Most of the costs of eradication activities are covered by UNICEF, Global 2000, bilateral agencies, NGOs and the countries themselves. WHO's role is limited to monitoring and surveillance of eradication and certification of eradication.[4]

The elimination of leprosy as a 'public health problem'

In 1991, The World Health Assembly committed the Organization to this Programme, to be completed by the year 2000 (Res.44.9). WHO considers that leprosy will no longer be a public health problem when the number of cases in a given country falls below one per 10 000 population. Globally, there has already been a significant 83 per cent decrease in the number of registered cases in the world, from 5.3 million in 1985 to under one million in 1995. Today, leprosy remains a public health problem in 60 countries or areas. Sixteen of these are rated the 'most endemic countries'.

By the beginning of 1996, about eight million patients had been cured with the WHO-recommended multidrug therapy (MDT). By mid-1996, the global coverage of MDT stood at over 90 per cent. The Global Plan for Action drawn by WHO and its collaborators envisages the identification and cure of nearly three million cases by the year 2000. This Plan had been recommended by the Hanoi Declaration adopted by an International Conference on the Elimination of Leprosy in July 1994.

WHO, through its Action Programme for the Elimination of Leprosy, oversees the quest for resources, monitors and evaluates the activities in each endemic country, and generally coordinates the progress towards elimination worldwide. It promotes the building up of national capabilities and encourages research for still more effective drugs.

WHO works in close collaboration with the member associations of the International Federation of Anti-Leprosy Associations, who work in the field with leprosy patients, and with the World Bank. Through the support of the Nippon Foundation of Japan, WHO supplies the drugs needed for MDT in blister packs in order to treat about 800 000 patients per year in some 25 countries.[5]

WHO's current programmes to control infectious diseases: a selection

The Expanded Programme on Immunization

WHO created its Expanded Programme on Immunization (EPI) in 1974, a global programme to immunize the children of the world against diphtheria, measles, poliomyelitis, tetanus, tuberculosis and whooping cough. EPI's objective was to reduce childhood morbidity and mortality through immunization, by making the best vaccines available and using them in the most effective manner. In 1994, EPI was integrated in the Global Programme for Vaccines and Immunization. From 1984 to 1993, EPI was financed almost equally by the regular budget – $58 million – and by extrabudgetary contributions – $60 million.[6]

In 1974, coverage for children under one year of age in developing countries was well below five per cent. Coverage rose to 50 per cent in 1987 for all vaccines except measles, and to 80 per cent in 1994, again with the exception of measles. The difficulty of implementing global immunization of children was shown by the fact that 80 per cent had already been reached in 1990, followed by a drop-off in 1991 and three subsequent years of no growth. Still, WHO estimates that in 1994 alone almost three million child deaths from the targeted diseases were prevented. While WHO provides leadership and technical guidance, UNICEF actively supports this Programme through advocacy, financial contributions, its operational work, providing vaccines and material for the cold chain.

The Children's Vaccine Initiative (CVI) was launched following the 1990 World Summit for Children. It includes WHO, UNICEF, UNDP, the World Bank and the Rockefeller Foundation as co-sponsors. A number of other public and private sector organizations are carrying out research programmes to improve the effectiveness and potency of vaccines.[7]

The Onchocerciasis Control Programme

Onchocerciasis (river blindness) is the world's second leading infectious cause of blindness, prevalent mainly in Africa. The Onchocerciasis Control Programme (OCP) was launched in 1974 covering seven, then 11 countries in West Africa, a combined population of about 30 million people. The Programme is jointly sponsored by WHO, the World Bank, UNDP and FAO, and is supported by a coalition of 22 donor countries and agencies. WHO acts as the Executive Agency, while the World Bank is responsible for mobilizing resources and administering the OCP Trust Fund. By the end of the century, it is estimated that the vector-control programme will have prevented almost 300 000 cases of blindness in the 11 participating countries, and opened 25 million hectares of fertile riverine land for resettlement and cultivation. OCP is scheduled to end by the year 2002. In June 1994, the World Bank approved funding for a new initiative, the African Programme for Onchocerciasis Control (APOC), to be implemented in the remaining 16 countries where onchocerciasis exists and which were not covered by OCP. In a new global strategy, onchocerciasis control will be based on yearly administration of single doses of ivermectin to affected populations. The drug is provided free of charge by Merck & Company. In 1994, the Programme was employing 200 WHO staff members in African countries, engaged mostly on a local basis, under the direction of a small team of international specialists and managers in Ouagadougou. Programme costs for the period 1974–94 were approximately $511 million.[8]

The Global Programme on AIDS

The WHO Global Programme on AIDS (GPA) was established in 1987. The Programme has been praised for providing leadership in mobilizing support for international and national AIDS prevention, care and support of 'persons living with HIV/AIDS' and promotion and coordination of research. GPA helped developing countries to plan and initiate activities to combat the pandemic. Over 160 national AIDS programmes were set up with WHO's financial and technical support. The dedication and exceptional contribution of GPA staff has been recognized by the World Health Assembly.[9]

The WHO Programme was replaced in January 1996 by a new Joint UN Programme on HIV/AIDS: its six co-sponsors are UNDP, UNICEF,

UNFPA, WHO, UNESCO and the World Bank. Its creation could only be seen as a public rebuff to WHO: it implied that WHO had not succeeded in being the 'directing and coordinating authority', mandated by its Constitution (Art. 2(a)), in this domain. A kinder and, in part, relevant interpretation is that 'WHO's technical base was too narrowly medical for it to deal effectively with AIDS prevention and control'.[10]

What is wrong with WHO?

In order to deal effectively at the international level with emerging and resurgent infectious diseases, besides other activities, WHO needs a clear mandate and clear priorities, achievable objectives, adequate technical, financial and human resources, dynamic leadership and a light and adaptable structure. According to critics, WHO is now lacking in some or most of these requirements.

The previous Director-General, Dr Mahler, a Danish national, put an unusually candid, Hamlet-like, question to Member States' delegates to the Fortieth World Health Assembly in May 1987:

> Is WHO to be the Organization you have decided it should be, the Organization that will lead the people of this world to health for all by the year 2000? Or is it to be merely a congregation of romanticists talking big and acting small; or just another international group of middlemen, giving pocket money to ministries of health and keeping a percentage for its own survival?[11]

A number of assessments of WHO's effectiveness have been made by independent groups.

The Nordic assessments

Established as a joint endeavour of the governments of Denmark, Finland, Norway and Sweden, the Nordic UN Project was completed in 1991. Its aim was to generate ideas as to how the Nordic countries, generous donors and traditionally supportive of development programmes, could make constructive contributions to the discussion on reform of the UN in the economic and social fields.[12]

Its final report noted that over the last few decades there had been a major change in the orientation of the work of the major specialized agences, FAO, ILO, UNESCO and WHO: the importance of their traditional normative (that is, standard-setting), research and information roles had been reduced and their operational activities in the form of technical cooperation with developing countries had greatly increased. However, the technical quality, as well as the speed and reliability of administration of agency-executed projects had declined significantly during the 1980s. The funding base of the agencies had gradually changed from predominantly regular budget funding to an increasing reliance on extrabudgetary funding, reflecting the growing emphasis in agency activities on technical cooperation.

The Nordic Project identified four basic problems facing UN operational activities: a problem of fragmentation due to a highly dispersed institutional structure leading to a multitude of agencies and bodies; a problem of mandate, whereby most agencies compete with one another and at times engage in overlapping and duplicative activities; a problem of resources due to a constantly eroding funding base; and finally a problem of marginalization due to the ever-increasing leadership role played by other multilateral organizations, in particular the Bretton Woods Institutions.

The Nordic report included the following recommendations with regard to the four specialized agencies: a strengthening of their normative role; restoration of their analytical capacity through clearer priority-setting for available resources and the termination of obsolete or irrelevant activities; a redefinition of their role in the provision of technical cooperation, reducing their role in the execution of projects, in particular at the national level and increasing their role in upstream activities such as sectoral analysis and advice; correction of the balance between regular budget and extrabudgetary resources to ensure that governing bodies have influence over all the agencies' activities.

A DANIDA Report of 1991 evaluated WHO's activities and effectiveness in Kenya, Nepal, Sudan and Thailand. The report confirmed the 'patently weak' analytical capacity of WHO in those countries, some difficulties in integrating headquarters-run programmes into the mainstream of national programmes, lack of a system of WHO priorities in the countries, and the undue concentration of WHO's management powers and resources in politicized Regional Offices, leaving no scope for an effectively functioning country office. Country offices, run by WHO Representatives, are left with mainly diplomatic and some administrative tasks, with inadequate professional capacity.

The report further noted that the role of WHO in the area of primary health care

> was found to be very limited, with other donors being lead agencies in relation to both field programmes and government policy advice.

The marginal role of WHO in relation to other donors was even found within traditional WHO programmes like the expanded programme on immunization in Nepal and Sudan, where UNICEF was the programme "carrying" donor in terms of both financial support and technical assistance to programme implementation.[13]

The Joint Inspection Unit report

In an unusually frank report on decentralization in WHO issued in 1993,[14] Inspectors E.-I. Daes and A. Daoudy made some hard-hitting criticisms and proposals. Among the criticisms:

- WHO's decentralized system is perceived by the donor community, as much as by WHO headquarters itself, as malfunctioning to the point of a fiducial credibility crisis;
- The overall picture is one of organizational fragmentation verging on disintegration by mode of operation. The consequences include hobbled strategic direction of the Organization as a whole, high operational costs and functional inefficiencies due above all to the virtual impossibility to synchronize and coordinate cross-programme processes throughout the Organization;
- Most donors prefer to deal directly with recipient government agencies, prudently bypassing WHO's regional and country structures. The same donors show a predilection for channelling resources through headquarters-based technical cooperation and vertical programmes.

The Inspectors recommended that WHO develop a system of priorities in order to concentrate its resources on a narrower range of critical programmes and to decentralize as many programmes as appropriate to the country level for support by other partners and WHO Representatives in agreement with the governments concerned. The Executive Board should 'revitalize' its management oversight authority over Regional Committees. Regional Directors should be appointed by the Executive Board upon nomination by the Director-General and no longer elected by their Regional Committee. They would then become 'technical managers' instead of politicized 'servants of their regional electorates'.

Finally, they recommended that the Executive Board initiate a comprehensive review of the functioning and structuring of WHO's technical programmes and another review of WHO staffing with the objective of reversing rising staffing costs and grade escalation.

British reports

A series of articles published in British health policy and medical periodicals between 1993 and 1995 provided another well-researched, critical assessment of WHO's performance and offered remedies.[15] According to these reports, WHO suffers from 'eradicationitis', which causes the distortion of emphasis from gradual horizontal integration to top-down vertical intervention. WHO Regional Offices are inefficient and bureaucratic, they duplicate expertise available at the headquarters in Geneva, and are too bound up in regional politics. Country offices are poorly funded, WHO Representatives are often political appointees with little enthusiasm, hampered by bureaucratic and remote Regional Offices. They lack expertise in research methodology and health systems management, skills needed by countries. They have no money to support specific projects, so they are marginalized in the donor community at country level. WHO has neither the mandate nor the means to implement its own programmes and WHO's fellowships programmes, run by the Regional Offices, have no strategy: politics rather than policies dictate what happens.

One of the conclusions of these studies was that WHO needed more effective leadership. The role of WHO should be clarified, priorities should be set and staff cut dramatically in Geneva and Regional Offices. 'The WHO cannot continue to try to do everything; instead of doing many of 120 things badly, it should do a dozen things well.'

As proposed by the Nordic report, the British reports suggest that WHO should, rather than eradicating more diseases, set standards on running health services and promoting health, providing advice to Member States, and speaking up for the many marginalized peoples of the world. They recommend that the power of the Director-General and the Regional Directors should be reduced. There should be more investment and training at country level. Staff should be recruited on merit rather than by election or political patronage. Budgets should be set in relation to the priorities and constantly reviewed. The final message for WHO was: 'change or die'.

To summarize these varied and not always compatible assessments and proposals, the remedies to WHO's ailments should be the following: (a) Clarify the role of WHO, set priorities, and focus on standard-setting and technical advice; (b) Reform WHO's structure, reduce the powers of Regional Offices, de-politicize Regional Directors, leave technical expertise to headquarters staff; (c) Strengthen country offices technically and financially, by appointing technically qualified and dedicated WHO Representatives, with more delegation of authority from Regional

Offices; (d) Cut down staff at headquarters and in Regional Offices, recruit staff on merit, not on patronage.

WHO's rivals

On its fiftieth anniversary in 1998 WHO found itself in direct competition, in its own domain, with other organizations and governments, at the global or at the regional level.[16] Some may 'rival' WHO in specific domains – MCH for UNICEF, family planning for UNFPA – or in overall programmes the World Bank, UNDP, the European Union. Some take more dynamic initiatives, some have a more visible and positive public image, some have more financial resources, some can provide the 'goods' more effectively and at lower cost.

In the UN system

In the UN family, UNICEF has a high profile in field operations such as mass immunization campaigns and emergency relief. From the late 1970s, UNICEF has assumed a strong advocacy role in the new Strategy of Health for All by the Year 2000 and primary health care. It collaborates with WHO in many programmes, including the immunization of children, polio eradication, and is a co-sponsor of UNAIDS. In contrast with WHO country offices, UNICEF field offices have a large degree of autonomy. UNICEF's country staff tend to be younger than WHO Representatives, more enthusiastic and vocationally trained.[17]

The World Bank created a Population, Health and Nutrition Department in 1980. Between 1981 and 1990 its expenditures for health rose from about $33 million to $263 million, with disbursements expected to exceed $1 billion by 2000 – more than the total WHO budget for 1996, including regular and extrabudgetary contributions. The Bank has developed public health expertise among its staff. The Bank is a major partner in WHO Programmes such as the Onchocerciasis Control Programme, the Special Programme for Research and Training in Tropical Diseases, and such joint programmes as UNAIDS and the Children's Vaccine Initiative.

UNDP is concerned with all aspects of development, including health. At the global level, UNDP is a co-sponsor, along with other organizations, of WHO programmes on tropical research on human reproduction and of joint programmes – UNAIDS and the Children's Vaccine Initiative. In 1992–3, its financial contribution to the WHO Voluntary Fund for Health Promotion was $41.2 million. Its expenditures for technical cooperation, excluding administrative costs, totalled $1204 million in 1993.[18] At country level, UNDP should coordinate technical advice and input from UN systems organizations. As decided by the UN General Assembly in 1989 and confirmed in 1991 (Res. 44/211 and 46/219), the UNDP resident coordinator should be the leader of the UN system multisectoral team. UNDP coordination role at country level, long resisted by WHO, may be imposed by Member States.

At its meeting in Lyon in June 1996, the Group of Seven prescribed that:

> Regular meetings of donors in each country should be organized to facilitate the exchange of information and the shaping of programmes according to the comparative advantages of each institution. Bilateral donors should be involved in this process. The resident UN Coordinator or the World Bank or regional bank representative could organize these meetings at regular intervals.[19]

While WHO has constantly insisted on its specific and separate role at country level, it will have no option but to become one of many participants in these meetings. UNFPA's 'leading role in the UN system in promoting population programmes' and its specific mandate in family planning should complement WHO's research and training activities in human reproduction, but could well overtake part of WHO's responsibilities in this field. Its expenditures reached $134.2 million in 1993.[20]

European rivals

Outside the UN system, the need for WHO to have Regional Offices has been questioned, particularly in Europe, where both the Council of Europe and the European Union have competence and programmes in public health. The Union, with substantial financial resources and political influence, is funding medical research and emergency relief. The Union has recently instituted a policy for the development of orphan drugs. It favours a more widespread use of generic drugs in order to reduce costs. The Union and its Members assist developing countries both bilaterally and multilaterally. Reorganization of health services, of pharmaceutical policy, of disease prevention and health promotion were included in its PHARE and TACIS programmes for the countries of central and eastern Europe and the newly independent states of the former USSR. Programmes on cancer, on AIDS and on other communicable diseases were designed specifically by the Union for these countries. Disease prevention and health protection were integrated into humanitarian operations carried out within the programme of the European Community Humanitarian Office (ECHO). A joint task force of the European Union and the USA has been set up to establish an effective, global, early-warning system and response network for communicable diseases which will collaborate with WHO and will encourage scientists from developing countries to work in European Union and US research programmes.

If its Members so decide, the European Union could well take over the full mandate of the WHO Regional Office, whose resources could be reallocated to programmes for developing countries. In the Americas, the WHO Regional Office is only a small part of the Pan-American Sanitary Bureau, which is the real political, technical and financial leader.

A US initiative

In May 1996, the Ministers of Health of Cyprus, Egypt, Israel, Jordan and the Palestinian Authority signed an agreement establishing a Middle East cancer consortium. The parties to the agreement are to collaborate on cancer research, epidemiology and treatment. The consortium was not initiated by WHO, but by the National Cancer Institute in the USA as part of the US efforts to promote peace in the Middle East.[21]

The role of non-governmental organizations

NGOs play a dynamic role in initiating, managing and/or supporting health programmes, in cooperation with WHO or independently. NGOs' contributions to the UN system to fund projects totalled $36 million in 1993: WHO was the recipient of about two-thirds of the contributions. Among the major contributors were Merck Sharp and Dohme Research, the Rockefeller and the Rotary Foundations, from the US, and the Japanese Sasakawa Health Trust Fund. As noted above, Rotary's PolioPlus programme provides operational and financial assistance to the WHO Polio Eradication Programme. Independently from WHO, the Johns Hopkins Program for International Education in Reproductive Health provides family-planning programmes in more than 40 countries. The Rockefeller Foundation is the main contributor to Inclen, the international clinical epidemiology network. The network provides training and financial support to mid-career professionals from developing countries in order to build up a critical mass of research expertise in medical schools.[22]

Another challenger to WHO's monopoly appeared in 1993 with the creation of the Council on Health Research for Development (COHRED). This NGO works with developing countries to strengthen their research capacity, to identify their major health problems and to find solutions which are most appropriate to them. COHRED supports the concept and practice of the Essential National Health Research (ENHR) strategy, with a country-specific focus. Its process involves scientists, policy- and decision-makers and community representatives. The bulk of its work takes place in countries under the oversight of an 18-member Board, with a small secretariat in Geneva. In 1996, from 40 to 60 countries were involved in the ENHR process. COHRED collaborates with UNDP, UNICEF, the World Bank, WHO, USAID, the EU, SIDA and NGOs. Its budget for 1996 was approximately $1.1 million.[23]

The WHO response to global change

In January 1992 the WHO Executive Board decided to undertake a review of WHO's response to the 'profound changes, – political, economic and social – ...affecting the world' through a Working Group appointed from among its members. Its final report was submitted in April 1993 (Doc. EB92/4). Its 47 recommendations were to be acted upon by the Director-General, the Executive Board itself, or a series of working partners.

The report expressed some justified fear that WHO's leadership on global health programmes and initiatives could be 'displaced' as other UN agencies or international bodies have increased their efforts to assume direction of specific health and environmental initiatives. According to an opinion poll of Member States conducted by the Working Group during the May 1993 Assembly, there was a need for WHO to strengthen its capabilities to provide technical cooperation in the areas of health policy formulation, planning, resource mobilization and infrastructure development for health care delivery, control of endemic diseases and assurance of a healthy overall environment. Often described as 'seven WHOs' (headquarters and the six Regional Offices), the Organization must avoid compartmentalization and fragmentation.

In January 1994 the Director-General created six internal 'development teams' as multidisciplinary groups set up to develop elements of policy, concepts or managerial tools in the following areas: WHO policy and mission, programme development and management, management and information systems, information and public relations, role of the WHO Representatives, personnel policy. However, the teams were composed of serving staff without input from external, independent consultants.

New units and activities

As an institutional response to the threat of new and re-emerging infectious diseases, the Director-General created in October 1995 the Division of Emerging, Viral and Bacterial Diseases Surveillance and Control. Its mission is 'to strengthen national and international capacity in the surveillance and control of communicable diseases which represent new, emerging or re-emerging public health problems, including the problem of antibiotic resistance, for which it will provide a timely and effective response'.

As a rapid response unit, the Division has the capacity to mobilize staff from both headquarters and Regional Offices, placing the teams on-site within 24 hours' notification of an outbreak, together with the supplies and equipment required to implement epidemic control measures. For instance, in the outbreak of Ebola haemorrhagic fever in Zaire, WHO staff from Geneva and Brazzaville arrived at the epidemic site within 24 hours of notification in Geneva, at the same time that the diagnosis of Ebola was confirmed at the WHO Collaborating Centre on Vital Haemorrhagic Fevers at CDC. WHO staff and nationals from Zaire set up a disease detection system and trained medical students in its operation so that all cases could be found and isolated. The outbreak was contained and its spread to Kinshasa, the capital city of two million inhabitants, was prevented.

WHO has established an information system (WHONET) to support the global surveillance of bacterial resistance to antimicrobial agents, with the participation of 177 laboratories in 31 countries or areas.

The Forty-Eighth Assembly has also requested the revision and updating of the International Health Regulations, with due regard to the evolution in the public health threat caused by the new or re-emerging infectious diseases.

In 1989, a Division of Emergency and Humanitarian Action had been created in Geneva, in order to coordinate the international response to emergencies and natural disasters in the health field, in cooperation with other UN agencies. However, it is more than doubtful that WHO would be unreservedly accepted by all other humanitarian organizations as the leader in such operations, with the authority to 'coordinate' their activities.

The Division's functions include the provision of emergency drugs and supplies, fielding of technical emergency assessment missions, expert advice to Member States on epidemiological surveillance, control of communicable diseases, public health information and health emergency training. Its main objective is to strengthen the national capacity of Member States to reduce the adverse health consequences of emergencies and disasters. During 1995, WHO assisted in relief efforts in 55 Member States, conducted emergency preparedness activities in 10, and cooperated in safety promotion and injury control in 11.[24]

Also in 1989, WHO launched a special initiative for intensified cooperation with countries and peoples in greatest need, called IWC, a poverty-oriented initiative. The Division of Intensified Cooperation with Countries (ICO) was made responsible for promoting and coordinating this programme in WHO. By August 1995, ICO was working with 26 countries. However, this headquarters-led programme seemed to conflict or overlap with Regional Offices' responsibilities. According to a report by an independent Study Team, IWC could be interpreted as either a redundancy or a compensatory initiative.[25]

Three priorities

In 1996, WHO proposed to the World Health Assembly three priorities for international action to combat infectious diseases during the following five years. The first priority is to complete unfinished business, namely to complete the eradication and elimination of diseases such as poliomyelitis, dracunculiasis, leprosy, measles, Chagas disease and onchocerciasis. This does not require a huge expenditure.

The second priority is to tackle old diseases such as tuberculosis and malaria which present new problems of drug and insecticide resistance. There is a need to remove infectious sources in the community and cure a high proportion of infectious cases, set up national and international epidemiological surveillance, and undertake research on treatment regimens and improved diagnostics, drugs and vaccines. Work is also needed on developing new and improved vaccines against measles, neonatal tetanus, bacterial meningitis, tuberculosis and other diseases.

The third priority is to take short-term and long-term action to combat newly emerging diseases. There is need for speedy action, research and a global surveillance programme.[26]

In a report submitted to the World Health Assembly in May 1996 (Doc. A49/11), the Director-General claimed that since WHO was set up in 1948 there has never been such an intensive effort over such a short period of time to introduce changes at all levels of the Organization. While the development teams involved more than 600 staff members at all WHO levels, the managerial and budgetary reform has *de facto* involved all programme staff. More than 90 documents went to the governing bodies, which responded with over 60 decisions and resolutions.

However, the same document, reporting on the 'implementation of recommendations on the WHO response to global change' was long on abstract generalities and future studies, leading to more reports, and short on specific achievements. Committees had been created within the Secretariat, the Global Policy Council, the Management Development Committee, composed of the Director-General and Regional Directors. They were to ensure, 'through a coordinated approach to programming, budgeting, monitoring and evaluation, that programme implementation at headquarters and at regional and country levels follows the global policy while respecting national priorities'. WHO's role at country level was to be clarified and redefined (in the future), budgetary reform was to be pursued, further improvements were to be made in programme planning and management, personnel policy would remain under continuous review, a programme management information system would be developed. But the report lacked substantive proposals on a new role and mandate for WHO, on programme priorities and on restructuring of Regional and country Offices.

Member States' criticisms and proposals – May 1996

At the World Health Assembly held in May 1996, the general mood of government delegates was not wholly condemnatory but often critical. A number of statements implied that real reform had not yet taken place and that the Director-General and his team still had to show that they were determined and capable of initiating substantial change in the Organization.

The US delegate affirmed that his country was deeply committed to WHO's success. However, the Organization 'must deepen its commitment to reform' and 'we must ensure strong, representative, and tough-minded leadership for WHO'. The Organization must concentrate its work on the global community's most urgent health problems. It must focus on what it does best: exerting global leadership in health, mobilizing global resources to respond to health emergencies, and giving countries the information, support, and other tools they need to effectively promote health and development.

The delegate from Brazil said that the structure, role and functions of WHO itself were in need of thorough review. WHO needed a more catalytic role, which should reinforce its technical, normative and information functions and encourage national leadership and self-reliance. For the delegate from Pakistan, WHO's celebrated successes in the fight against communicable diseases were under threat. A new global strategy was needed, which would focus on surveillance and control of infectious diseases and the development of new and effective drugs. The Dutch delegate said that in setting priorities among communicable diseases, the burden imposed by each disease and the cost-effectiveness of intervention – established by research – should be the criteria used. WHO should pay particular attention to the major killers such as diarrhoeal diseases, respiratory infections, tuberculosis and malaria, and new initiatives were needed in that regard. There was need for a speedy response to outbreaks of communicable diseases, to prevent potential epidemics. To achieve that response, an early warning system and clear guidelines for outbreak management were crucial. The Organization would have to prove that it was a key player in the field of communicable diseases.[27]

Besides formal government statements in the World Health Assembly, a number of countries and private groups continued, and expanded on, the Nordic Project of 1991.

In 1994, the governments of Australia, Norway and the UK (the Oslo Group) sponsored a study of extrabudgetary funds in WHO. The governments of Sweden, Canada and Italy then joined the Group. The Potantico retreat entitled 'Enhancing the Performance of International Health Institutions' was held in New York in February 1996 by the Rockefeller Foundation, the US Social Science Research Council and the Harvard School of Public Health. In April 1996, the Dag Hammarskjöld Foundation organized a meeting on 'Global Health Cooperation in the 21st Century and the Role of the UN System'.

This heavy concentration on the issues of international health reflected in part the frustration of these governments and groups with WHO's uneven efforts at self-reform. Their contributions should help governments decide on how WHO, and its UN partners, should be reformed: which tasks should be assumed by which organization, with what resources.

Conclusion

WHO is in a new world of high competition: if they want 'their' organization to regain its title of recognized leader in international public health, and not only to survive, its Member States, governing bodies and the Director-General have to show resolve and tangible results in their still uncoordinated and, for some critics, half-hearted efforts towards reform.

WHO has important assets. It is the only global international organization in its domain, in which all countries, rich and poor, are represented. Its legitimacy is based on an international, objective, impartial consensus on health policies, a consensus which cannot be achieved in international politics. WHO has a broad base of regional and national representation through its Regional and country offices. More than 1000 Collaborating Centers and 181 NGOs maintain working relations with WHO.

Most observers recognize that WHO's comparative advantage *vis-à-vis* other health-oriented organizations is its global role in policy formulation and development, both for common global needs and support of technical cooperation with developing countries. WHO's research activities in its co-sponsored, large programmes are examples of 'centres of excellence'. The indirect benefits achieved by other organizations using WHO's 'products' (scientific findings and publications, norms and standards, policies, strategies, monitoring and evaluation capacity) have been considerable. An association with WHO provides a respected legitimacy to other organizations in WHO-approved joint programmes. WHO managers have understood the absolute need to cooperate with other governmental, intergovernmental and non-governmental organizations, not only for financial reasons, but also to broaden the impact of their programmes, to increase their effectiveness and to enlist more popular support for the work of their Organization.

A more general, encouraging, asset is that most Member States, for varying reasons, support the Organization, although most industrialized countries want WHO to renovate itself and become more 'cost-effective'. Even the US, the major and more aggressive critic of the UN system, has maintained its commitment to WHO's success, a commitment which is, however, conditional on its reform.

Reform what? WHO's weaknesses have been identified: a refusal to set effective priorities, leading to an overextended programme of dispersed, poorly financed projects – bureaucratic and politicized Regional Offices, which duplicate better expertise available at headquarters, lack of effectiveness at country level, and leadership and management problems.

Who should conduct WHO's reform ? Bureaucracies do not reform themselves. The *WHO Response to Global Change* initiated in 1993 has been criticized for its apparent lack of substantial results, one reason being that its process is almost exclusively driven internally by its secretariat, without real input, direction and control by its governing bodies.

It is likely that the new WHO will be leaner and will focus on what it does best: global, inter-regional activities, its normative role, formulation of public health policy, promotion and coordination of research, development of new technologies, methodologies, vaccines, medicaments, global and national health statistics.

WHO should improve its capacity to deal with emerging and resurgent infectious diseases by improving global epidemiological surveillance. WHO should reinforce its participation in the setting up of the global early warning system and response network for communicable diseases being designed by the European Union and the US, through a maximum use of WHO Collaborating Centers. The resources available to the new WHO rapid-response unit should be increased. Research on infectious disease agents, their evolution, the vectors of disease spread and control methods, vaccines and drug development should also be encouraged.

WHO headquarters should retain its key role in initiating and monitoring global immunization campaigns, as well as global disease eradication and control programmes. Technical units together with international expert groups should retain their current responsibilities in this domain: assessing the technical soundness and operational feasibility of such programmes; defining strategy, policies and timed objectives; submitting their proposals to the World Health Assembly for approval; creating alliances for the financing and implementation of programmes. WHO should continue to serve as the global technical reference, and should be responsible for the monitoring and evaluation of the activities. Operational responsibilities would be mainly assumed by UNICEF, bilateral agencies and NGOs, better qualified for this role. Member States and other donors should provide adequate financing of approved programmes.

WHO staff have the competence and capacity to take up these new challenges, but they need a clear signal from Member States, governing bodies and from their own leadership that a real reform of the Organization has started.

* The author has written this contribution in a personal capacity: views and conclusions are his own responsibility. They do not necessarily represent WHO's position, nor do they commit the Organization in any way.

Notes

1 L. J. Bruce-Chwatt, 'Worldwide Malaria Eradication: a Dream or Reality?'
   WHO Features (August 1988); Javed Siddiqi, *World Health and World Politics*

(London: Hurst, 1995), Part III; *WHO Fact Sheet* No. 94, 12 March 1996, 'Malaria'.

2 See the *Final Report of the Global Commission for the Certification of Smallpox Eradication*, WHO, 1988.

3 *WHO Fact Sheet* No. 114, 'Global Polio Eradication, The 1995 Progress Report', May 1996.

4 *WHO Fact Sheet* No. 98, December 1995.

5 *WHO Fact Sheet* No. 101, May 1996.

6 Extra contributions came mainly from the Nordic countries, the Netherlands, Japan, Rotary International, Australia and the USA. See Doc. WHO/EPI/GEN/94.1, Section 11.

7 *WHO Press Releases* WHO/73, October 1995; WHO/43, June 1996.

8 *WHO Fact Sheet* No. 95, November 1995.

9 WHO Doc. EB95/48, January 1995; Res. WHA49.27, May 1996.

10 Fiona Godlee, 'WHO in Retreat: is it Losing its Influence?' *British Medical Journal*, 309 (1994) 3 December p. 1494.

11 Doc. WHA40/DIV/4, 5 May 1987.

12 Nordic UN Project, *Perspective on Multilateral Assistance* (Stockholm: Almdqvist & Wiksell International, 1991).

13 DANIDA, 'Effectiveness of Multilateral Agencies at Country Level: WHO in Kenya, Nepal, Sudan and Thailand' (Copenhagen: Danida, 1991).

14 UN Doc. JIU/REP/93/2 (Part III), 'Decentralization of Organizations within the UN System' (Geneva, 1993).

15 Among these, G. Walt, 'WHO Under Stress: Implications for Health Policy', *Health Policy*, 24 (1993) pp. 125–44; Fiona Godlee, a series of articles on WHO, *British Medical Journal*, 309–310 (November 1994–March 1995), ending with Editor Richard Smith's conclusion, *British Medical Journal*, 310 (4 March 1995) pp. 543–4.

16 Kelley Lee, 'Who Does What in Health ? Mandates within the UN System', *UN & Health Briefing Note*, International Health Policy Programme, London School of Hygiene and Tropical Medicine, No. 1 (September 1995); see also Fiona Godlee's series of articles on WHO, op. cit.

17 Fiona Godlee, *British Medical Journal*, 309 (1994) p. 1637.

18 WHO Doc. A47/19 Add.1, Annex, 11 April 1994, p. 4; and UN Doc. DP/1994/40/Add.1, 28 September 1994, para. 79.

19 See *International Documents Review*, 7 (24), (24–28 June 1996).

20 UN Doc. DP/1994/40/Add.1, para. 74.

21 WHO Doc. A49/A/SR/1, 21 May 1996: statements of the delegates of Italy, France and Israel, pp. 3, 5, 11.

22 Richard L. Sullivan, 'Training Across International Borders', *Training and Development* (June 1995) pp. 55–7; Fiona Godlee, *British Medical Journal*, 310 (1995) p. 111.

23 *COHRED Progress Report 1995*.

24 WHO Doc. A49/6 of 29 February 1996; *WHO Fact Sheet* No. 90, July 1995.

25 'Cooperation for Health Development – Extrabudgetary Funds in the World Health Organization', May 1995, Australia, Norway, United Kingdom, Appendix 4C.

26 WHO Doc. A49/3, 25 March 1996, p. 13.

27 WHO Doc. A49/A/SR/1, 2 and 3, 21 and 22 May 1996.

11

Knowledge, Information and Intergovernmental Cooperation

Donald A. Henderson

Introduction

Successfully meeting the global challenge of new and emerging infections requires that mechanisms be established or expanded to identify rapidly and to characterize the offending agents. Controlling the threat will necessitate the participation of research establishments and scientists, as well as national and international institutions prepared to respond in a timely manner. There is now, however, a substantial gap between what is needed and what is available with regard to mechanisms, institutions and expertise for early detection, definition and control of potential threats. There are limitations, as well, in the capacity of existing international structures to mobilize a broad coherent response. The problem is further exacerbated by national political sensitivities and a reluctance sometimes to report, even if recognized, the occurrence of infectious disease outbreaks which might be of international concern.

Nations in both the industrialized and the developing world, individually and collectively, are today ill-prepared technically to cope with the new microbial challenges. Expertise in all aspects of the infectious disease field – be it clinical, epidemiological, research or diagnostic – has steadily eroded over the past 40 years. Although a modest rejuvenation has occurred in certain of these disciplines coincident with a mobilization to deal with the HIV pandemic, only modest efforts have been devoted to diseases other than HIV. National reporting and surveillance systems which might serve as sentinel alerts are woefully inadequate to non-existent, and recognition of the potential gravity of the new and emerging microbial threats is still limited.

In designing needed new responses, it is important to appreciate both the present status and relevant past experiences in dealing internationally with infectious disease problems as well as to understand the administrative and political developments leading to today's problems. These are elaborated upon in this chapter following which a brief summary is presented of future actions which might be taken.

The demise of expertise and surveillance in the infectious disease field

Throughout the industrialized world, there has been a pervasive and growing complacency that infectious diseases are effectively past history, at least in the well-sanitized environments inhabited by national policy-makers. There is cause for this complacency. After World War II, standards of living steadily increased; nutrition improved; and clean water and indoor sanitary systems became all but universal. Along with a cornucopia of new antibiotics and vaccines a great many of the previously common childhood illnesses were eliminated and many of the bacterial, mycotic and parasitic infections could be treated and cured.

The primary interests of both the health care and medical research communities began to shift to those diseases which were the principal causes for hospitalization and commanded the lion's share of medical care time and expense – such as chronic cardiac and pulmonary disease, cancer, arthritis and diabetes. Priority was given to expanding rapidly a network of 'sickness care' establishments – hospitals and clinics, to providing specialized professional training to staff these and to supporting the relevant research agendas.

Gradually, the budgets and competence of public health establishments declined. Interest in disease prevention and community-based public health measures such as immunization, were subordinated or ignored in favor of more dramatic although increasingly costly procedures including ever more elaborate surgical and diagnostic interventions, organ transplantation, cancer chemotherapy and radiation, and renal dialysis.

A growing confidence that the infectious diseases were of marginal importance led inexorably to fewer professionals seeking training in the clinical, epidemiological and laboratory aspects of the infectious diseases and gradually both laboratories and training centers closed. In the developing countries, this process was accelerated by the growing number of countries becoming independent states and the decision by former colonial powers to diminish or to cease support in those countries of medical research and training centers, most of which were concerned with infectious diseases. Philanthropic institutions tended to do the same.

Infectious diseases in the developing world remained the overwhelmingly dominant problem but newly independent nations had too few resources to sustain the existing centers. Such investments as could be made were largely assigned to sickness care hospitals in capital cities. Disease surveillance likewise deteriorated. The effectiveness of surveillance systems is directly proportional to the extent that the data are actively used and to the extent that those submitting the data understand their importance. So long as concerns about infectious illnesses remained high and health departments had the capacity to deal with them, there was an impetus to collect and analyze data on a concurrent basis. With early warning, outbreaks of polio or diphtheria, for example, could be countered by vaccination; food-borne outbreaks would be detected and problems corrected; vector control could serve to abort outbreaks of mosquito-borne encephalitis. Such surveillance systems thus were used not only for program operation but for strategic planning and resource allocation as well. However, with the balance of concerns of the health care system shifting from public health to sickness care, from concern about the overall health of the community to the care and rehabilitation of individual sick patients, interest in community-based data waned as did its quality.

The detection and reporting of cases

Data regarding health and illness in the industrialized countries are surprisingly incomplete and seldom current while in developing countries, data on most diseases represent little more than the crudest of approximations. Few professionals, even in the medical field itself, appreciate how little current, comprehensive, accurate information on human health is routinely collected. This is in sharp contrast to the status of such as the agricultural sector, for example, where in many countries substantial data are routinely collected and analyzed. The data include a wide variety of information, such as the numbers of farm animals and their productivity, numbers of acres of different crops grown and their yield, illnesses and causes of death of animals. The diligence with which these data are collected, analyzed and published is usually attributed to the fact that such data bear on strategic planning decisions, on program operations and on resource allocations and payments. The fact that comparably complete and current data on human morbidity and mortality do not exist is moot testimony to the fact that the prevalence and trends in disease incidence have little to do with the setting of priorities or the allocation of resources in health systems.

The existing reporting systems for human disease take many different forms, the most common consisting of annual or monthly, seldom weekly, reports from hospitals and sometimes clinics purported to enumerate the number of cases of some 25–50 specified diseases seen during the reporting period. The limitations and flaws of such systems are legion. In third world countries, clinics and hospitals are typically understaffed with only the most rudimentary, manual record-keeping systems and limited to nonexistent laboratory capabilities. Cases which are reported are customarily those whose diagnoses are entered into some sort of daily ledger after a few minutes' contact with a physician or health aide, usually without benefit of supporting laboratory information. A patient with an acute febrile illness, for example, might equally well be diagnosed as having any of a number of diseases including malaria, dengue, yellow fever or influenza. Continued observation over several days as to the course of illness as well as laboratory studies would serve to narrow the range of diagnostic possibilities, but pressed for time and with limited recourse to a laboratory, health care staff can do little but offer a best-guess diagnosis. In industrialized countries, one anticipates a better performance than this from academic health centers and larger hospitals but doubtfully much better in many poorer socioeconomic areas and in rural communities.

The problem of data gathering is further exacerbated by the fact that comparatively few health units which are expected to report, actually do so. Seldom do the statistical offices which are responsible for collecting reports actively take steps to assure timely and complete reporting. Thus, in Latin America and the Caribbean prior to the 1985 launch of the polio eradication campaign, all data on disease incidence came from approximately 500 hospitals which usually submitted reports once each month.[1] What proportion of the actual total of cases of various diseases which these facilities might have seen and reported is unknown. Various estimates suggest perhaps one per cent to five per cent for a serious disease such as acute paralytic poliomyelitis to as little as one-tenth to one one-hundredth this proportion for less serious and distinctive infections. Least well reported are those illnesses which are seen primarily by local physicians or healers not working in a hospital or which may not be brought to anyone for medical care, such as often happens with cases of measles. Eventually, in Latin America, a network of 20 000 health units was developed which reported weekly and this, it was determined, was able to detect virtually all cases of acute flaccid paralysis, albeit a somewhat lower proportion of neonatal tetanus cases and a substantially lower proportion of measles cases.

Another indication of the deficiencies of conventional reporting systems is available from experiences during the smallpox eradication campaign.[2] Of all the infectious diseases, smallpox was the one which should have been the best reported. Under terms of the International Health Regulations (IHR) to which all countries are signatory, countries were obligated to report promptly to the World Health Organization (WHO) all cases of smallpox occurring within their borders. This was one of only five diseases to which these regulations then pertained. Smallpox cases typically were severe and likely to be seen by hospitals and other health care providers. Moreover, the cases had a distinctive rash which permitted ready diagnosis without the need for laboratory studies. After the program began, it was possible to develop estimates of the true incidence of the disease and to compare these with the numbers of cases actually reported. Using population-based surveys, the proportion of persons with the characteristic residual scars of smallpox could be ascertained and from this information, it was possible to estimate the average annual numbers of cases. It was found that when the programme began in most countries, not more than one per cent to two per cent of all cases were then actually being reported. Although this was a situation which prevailed some 25 years ago, personal observation suggests that the quality of the systems is little better today.

Such unrecognized deficiencies in data have implications for health policy and resource allocation. Ethiopia is a case in point. It was the last endemic country to begin a smallpox eradication program, reluctantly doing so in 1971. Smallpox was considered not to be a problem, only 169 cases having been reported in 1969 and 722 cases in 1970. With the advent of the smallpox programme, a rudimentary reporting and surveillance system began to function in 1971 and although covering only part of the country, 26 329 cases were documented that year, a figure estimated to be perhaps 10 per cent of all cases which actually occurred. Not surprisingly, the interest of government in the program increased significantly after the magnitude of the problem became apparent. Similar experiences have been repeatedly documented for other diseases and in many different countries.

Delays in recognizing infectious diseases are not restricted to the developing countries. In the United States, a serious pneumonic illness called legionnaires' disease was first identified in 1976 and the responsible organism isolated.[3] Later, it was discovered that sporadic cases had actually occurred as early as 1947[4] and that there had been at least three other outbreaks extending over 20 years.[5] Similarly, toxic shock syndrome was not recognized until 1980, but afterwards cases could be documented to have occurred as early as 1960.

The stark fact is that ongoing, reasonably complete and reliable data with regard to the overall incidence of most diseases and the status of the health of populations as a whole are at best incomplete or essentially nonexistent in all countries. That situation could change. With growing concerns universally about constraining health care costs and the implicit need for strategic planning and alternative allocations of resources, data collection systems are beginning to receive more attention.

Response to outbreaks of disease

However inadequate reporting systems may be, the occurrence of unusually large numbers of infectious disease cases, especially when severe, are even now reported periodically by health care providers whatever the status of established reporting systems. With early, competent investigation and control of such outbreaks, more serious and widespread epidemics can sometimes be averted. However, few countries are suitably staffed or administratively structured to cope with such problems.

The investigation of disease outbreaks requires special, presently scarce, epidemiological skills no less than a heart bypass operation, for example, requires surgical skills. Although the public and professionals alike would be horrified to have an epidemiologist performing open-heart surgery, untrained medical staff are frequently assigned to undertake outbreak investigation and control. The results are frequently deplorable.

The United States and the United Kingdom, with respectively, the Centers for Disease Control and Prevention (CDC) and the Public Health Laboratory Service (PHLS), employ public health professional staff, including epidemiologists and microbiologists, who are on call to respond promptly to infectious disease outbreaks or other problems. Similar institutions and strategies are beginning to be developed by a number of countries in Europe as well as countries as diverse as Mexico, Thailand, Taiwan and Saudi Arabia. The result in these countries is that health staff, wherever situated, know that there is available competent help which could promptly respond to provide assistance. As experience has shown, when there is a prompt response to such a request, health staff are more likely to report outbreaks, thus bringing problems to light at an earlier time and when they are more manageable.

An outbreak response program such as this presumes an openness in communication and a willingness to deal with infectious disease outbreaks and problems objectively and scientifically. Governments, for a number of reasons, do not always choose to be so forthright in dealing with epidemic problems, with all too often adverse consequences for themselves and their neighbors. A classic illustration of this occurred in 1970 when smallpox was introduced into Iran in November of that year and began to spread.[6] The government, then preparing for major national celebrations and believing that an outbreak such as this would reflect adversely on the country, reported no cases despite the provisions of the IHR. Likewise, the government officially denied the presence of smallpox when WHO queried the validity of rumors which came from visitors to Iran and from the diplomatic community. Over 22 months, smallpox spread across Iran and later into Iraq, Syria and Yugoslavia. It was discovered eventually that at least 6000–8000 cases had occurred. Because of secrecy, it had been difficult for government health staff to detect and control new outbreaks. Meanwhile, more than 51 million vaccinations were performed, initially with substandard vaccine, before control was achieved. Early reporting of the problem, use of international expertise and fully potent vaccine could readily have stopped spread within six to eight weeks.

Governments have likewise suppressed reports of cholera cases, fearing that neighboring governments might invoke trade sanctions. Also, certain vacation resort areas, as a policy, deny the presence of any infectious diseases whatsoever.

Suppression of reports of disease outbreaks seems gradually to be waning, coincident with greater sophistication of government officials and the increasing willingness of countries with special expertise to make available needed help when asked. However, even as recently as 1996, we find in the United Kingdom a reluctance and an inexplicable and protracted delay in making public available basic data regarding cases of the human form of spongiform encephalopathy and an extended exclusion from the investigations by staff from its excellent Public Health Laboratory Service which was established specifically to deal with human health threats of this type.[7]

Finally, it must be noted that there is, on the part of governments and many scientists as well, a misplaced complacency regarding the probabilities of experiencing serious outbreaks due either to a new or emergent microbial infection or perhaps through the use by terrorists of a biological weapon. That complacency has been shaken, to some degree, by the development of the HIV pandemic. Even so, this effect has been mitigated, in part, by the fact that the epidemic developed over years, rather than weeks or months and that the majority of the victims acquired infection as a result of behaviors in which the majority of the population is thought not to engage. Biological terrorism, while understandable as a theoretical possibility, is regularly dismissed as unworthy of further concern on the grounds of it being morally reprehensible and because it has not been a documented reality since before 1940.

International leadership

The global repercussions implicit in the emergence of new infections demand international leadership and response of a different character than has heretofore been in evidence. Needed is cooperation in rapid information exchange, in the development of a surveillance structure for case detection, in characterizing new threats, and in the development of relevant research agendas.

A number of initiatives have now been started. The earliest and most important was comprehensive review of the problem in 1992 with specific recommendations for action proposed by an expert group under the auspices of the Institute of Medicine of the United States National Academy of Sciences.[8] This provided the basis for a detailed CDC plan to strengthen surveillance programmes[9] and that plan matured into a US government interagency action plan.[10] New allocations of funds have been earmarked for program activities. The Pan American Health Organization[11] and WHO[12] have reflected the principal components of the US plan in a broader global strategy and WHO has established a new unit charged with the responsibility for mobilizing and coordinating resources to respond to a challenge. At the Halifax Summit in 1995, the major industrialized countries formally recognized the problem in adopting a pilot program called 'Toward a Global Health Network'. Finally, on 12 June 1996, US Vice President Gore announced a new presidential policy calling for improved domestic and international surveillance, prevention and response measures to emerging infectious diseases and directed the relevant government agencies to work with other nations and international organizations to establish a global system.[13]

The common elements in the various plans have been summarized as follows:

- Strengthen international surveillance networks to detect, control and reduce emerging diseases
- Improve international capabilities to respond to disease outbreaks with adequate medical and scientific expertise and resources

- Strengthen international research efforts on emerging diseases
- Improve the public health infrastructure – laboratories, research facilities, and communications links
- Develop better international standards and guidelines[14]

The analyses and basic directions which are reflected in the various plans are reasonable but what are the prospects for the initiatives maturing into structures and operational modalities which will be fully responsive to the needs? Neither past history nor trends in recent events offer a great deal of encouragement.

The longest standing international effort to deal cooperatively with infectious disease problems is embodied in the implementation of WHO's International Health Regulations (IHR).[15] These regulations are now being rewritten but as they currently stand, they apply to only three diseases – plague, cholera and yellow fever. They provide for specific procedures to be followed in notification of the diseases as well as for prevention and control measures to be taken to prevent international spread. They also detail sanitary conditions, health facilities and personnel that should be available in seaports and airports, what maximum measures national health authorities may institute to protect their territories from the disease in question on departure, between ports of departure and arrival, and upon arrival. The regulations also stipulate certain measures to be followed in transport of goods, cargoes, luggage and mails.

Whatever the concern about the spread of these diseases across national borders, it is widely agreed that the regulations have proved generally to be of limited value. Although the regulations are binding on all member states when approved by the World Health Assembly, every country has the right to reject such provisions as it may wish, and many selectively do so. Moreover, there is no legal action which WHO can take to compel compliance with the regulations. Thus, if a member state wishes to suppress information about a disease, there is little WHO can do other than to exercise moral and scientific suasion to encourage compliance. WHO's ability to exert such leadership has been compromised over recent years as it has become increasingly politicized and its expertise has eroded.

A no less serious problem is the availability of resources. With fiscal economy being a lead agenda item in most industrialized countries, support for foreign assistance programs and international organizations has come under considerable pressure. Although foreign assistance allocations are small proportionate to total government budgets, they nevertheless are often viewed by policy-makers as being able to be reduced with little political consequence. To secure adequate support and financing for a new programs is predictably difficult under such circumstances. The likelihood that WHO might re-evaluate priorities to give greater weight to the new challenges seems remote. The organization is already deeply engaged in scaling back activities to cope with a budget crisis engendered primarily by a failure of the United States government to pay on time its agreed obligations.

The future

The potential challenge, the threat, posed by new or emerging infections should be motivation enough for nations and international organizations to address the problem aggressively, assigning such resources as are necessary and, as appropriate, reshaping international institutions to be responsive to the collective need. This seems not unreasonable given the reality of a worst-case scenario which places at stake the essential fabric of civilization as we know it. But will there be the needed commitment?

The fundamental building blocks for a global system must necessarily consist of units, primarily hospitals or clinics, which are capable of detecting and reporting unusual cases or constellations of cases.[16] Establishing such a network will require the strengthening of both clinical and laboratory competence in a substantial number of hospital centers and the linking of these centers with national public health expertise, with international organizations and with specialized international centers with infectious disease expertise. Additional resources and provisions for training will also be essential but, to date, little has been said about these needs or where the requisite support might come from.

For such a network to function effectively will require the full participation of each of its units in active surveillance programs, specifically the regular (weekly) submission of specified data to a national, eventually international center, the concurrent evaluation of these data and the feedback of the interpreted material to participant centers and others as a guide to future activities. Experience has shown that without the stimulus of ongoing interaction between reporting units and central program staff, systems quickly disintegrate and communications links are broken or forgotten.

A very difficult question, and one not yet resolved, is what basic data might best be routinely collected by all participant units which might serve as an alert to the occurrence of a new or emergent infection. One possible useful measure which is under consideration is a compilation of the number of non-traumatic deaths occurring weekly among those between the ages of perhaps five and 50 years of age. It is known that non-traumatic deaths within this age range are comparatively uncommon and thus, a notable increase in deaths might provide a useful, albeit crude alert signal indicating the need for special investigations. Had such a system been in place in past years, it is almost certain that the AIDS epidemic would have been detected one to two decades earlier; and similarly, would have provided an early alert for such as the swine flu epidemic of 1919, for epidemics of yellow fever, for Lassa fever and Ebola virus epidemics. All of these have been associated with notably high rates of mortality, especially in young adults.

In exploration of this hypothesis, US investigators in four states decided to look at all deaths occurring in 1992 among individuals between one and 49 years which were unexplained deaths due to possible infectious causes in previously healthy persons.[17] Comparatively few deaths were expected. To everyone's surprise, 744 such deaths were recorded in a population of 8.3 million persons. Follow-up studies are in progress. However, once again, a dramatic illustration is presented of how little is presently known about causes of mortality in the human population. It is also of note that the analysis was conducted on 1992 figures, already several years old, but the most recent year for which complete mortality data were available for the US.

In the meantime, efforts have begun to link widely by Internet various international centers which are collaborating in the investigation of different diseases, and a new journal, *Emerging Infectious Diseases*, has been launched by CDC.

The scientific community and the press have made gratifying progress in educating politicians and a broad public about the problem and the needs. However, further efforts are required in all countries. Time and effort will be required. In the past, the voice of respected international health leadership, especially in WHO and UNICEF, has been extremely valuable and, hopefully, respected professionals will assume that role again.

A number have proposed that collaboration in dealing with these problems be mandated rather than voluntary, specifically hoping for some form of legally binding treaty which might confront the problems of suppression of information and lack of cooperation by some WHO member states. It would seem unlikely that efforts of this sort would be well received, if for no other reason than the disappointing results to date in endeavoring to implement the International Health Regulations. What is often overlooked, however, is the degree of international cooperation which has been possible in any number of programs when WHO has exhibited professional competence and leadership in discharging its responsibilities. This continues to be exemplified most clearly in WHO's regional office for the Americas, the Pan American Health Organization. Such should be possible globally.

For the foreseeable future, then, progress in preparing an adequate response will most likely be dependent on voluntary national initiatives and networks of scientists interested in the problems and communicating by Internet while practical experience is gained in dealing with a variety of exigencies as they appear.

In the meantime, we must hope that none of the new or emerging infections assumes a highly transmissible, seriously lethal form which demands a more urgent response.

Notes

1 D. A. Henderson and C. A. deQuadros, 'The Eradication of Poliomyelitis', *Vaccines 95* (Cold Spring Harbor, NY: Cold Spring Harbor Press, 1995) pp. 413–22.

2 F. Fenner, D. A. Henderson, I. Arita, A. Jezek and I. D. Ladnyi, *Smallpox and Its Eradication* (Geneva: World Health Organization, 1988).

3 J. E. McDade, C. C. Shepard, D. W. Fraser et al., 'Isolation of a Bacterium and Demonstration of its Role in Other Respiratory Diseases', *New England Journal of Medicine*, 297 (1977) pp. 1197–203.

4 J. E. McDade, D. J. Brenner and F. M. Bogeman, 'Legionnaires' Disease Bacterium Isolated in 1947', *Annual of International Medicine*, 90 (1979) pp. 659–61.

5 M. T. Osterholm, T. D. Y. Chin, D. O. Osborne et al., 'A 1957 Outbreak of Legionnaires' Disease Associated with a Meat Packing Plant', *American Journal of Epidemiology*, 117 (1983) pp. 60–7; S. B. Thacker, J. V. Bennett, T. F. Tsai et al., 'An Outbreak in 1965 of Severe Respiratory Illness Caused by the Legionnaires' Disease Bacterium', *Journal of Infectious Disease*, 138 (1970) pp. 512–19; T. H. Glick, M. B. Gregg, B. Berman et al., 'Pontiac Fever: an Epidemic of Unknown Etiology in a Health Department', *American Journal of Epidemiology*, 107 (1978) pp. 149–60.

6 Fenner, Henderson et al., *Smallpox and Its Eradication*, op. cit.

7 S. R. Palmer, 'The BSE Crisis – An Assessment', *Eurohealth*, 2 (1996) pp. 3–4.

8 Institute of Medicine, *Emerging Infections* (Washington, DC: National Academy Press, 1992).

9 Centers for Disease Control and Prevention, *Addressing Emerging Infectious Disease Threats: a Prevention Strategy for the United States* (Atlanta: Department of Health and Human Services, 1994).

10 National Science and Technology Council, Committee on Science, Engineering and Technology: Working Group on Emerging and Re-Emerging Infectious Diseases, *Infectious Diseases – a Global Threat* (Washington, DC: CISET document, 1995).

11   D. B. Epstein (1995) 'Recommendations for a Regional Strategy for the Pre-
     vention and Control of Emerging Infectious Diseases in the Americas', *Emer-
     ging Infectious Diseases*, 1 (1995) pp. 103–5.
12   World Health Assembly, 'Communicable Diseases Prevention and Control:
     New, Emerging and Reemerging Infectious Diseases', WHO Doc. WHA
     48.13. (Geneva: WHO, 1995).
13   White House, 'Vice President Announces Policy on Infectious Diseases: New
     Presidential Policy Calls for Coordinated Approach to Global Issue'. Press
     release, 12 June 1996.
14   D. P. Fidler, 'Globalization, International Law and Emerging Infectious Dis-
     eases', *Emerging Infectious Diseases* 2 (1996) pp. 77–82.
15   World Health Organization, 'The Revision of the International Health Regu-
     lations, *Weekly Epidemiological Record*, 71 (1996) pp. 233–5.
16   D. A. Henderson, 'Surveillance Systems and Intergovernmental Cooperation',
     in S. S. Morse (ed.), *Emerging Viruses* (New York: Oxford University Press,
     1993) pp. 283–9.
17   B. A. Perkins, J. M. Flood, R. Danila et al., *Emerging Infectious Diseases,* 2
     (1996) pp. 47–53.

12
Surveillance, Eradication and Control: Successes and Failures[*]

William Foege

The successes and failures of disease eradication and control are well known; rather than highlight them, it is more instructive to consider the implications of these experiences. I will focus on six lessons that I think require examination, and then suggest steps that we might take.

The first is the absolute importance of problem definition. Part of this, of course, is surveillance, but surveillance is like grandparents – there is no substitute. It is so important it has to be a priority, and when we ask how much money to put into surveillance, the answer is 'enough'.

In the United States, our history is fairly recent. It is only in the last fifty years that we have had national surveillance for any single disease. That may come as a surprise to many. It was not until 1950 that we had the first surveillance program, which was for malaria. It found that we had no malaria. Malaria had quietly disappeared in the 1940s and we did not know it. Lots of people in the South still went to the doctor with fever, were treated for malaria and got better, and that perpetuated the idea that we still had malaria. It was not until people went out trying to get blood smears to find out what kind of malaria was prevalent that we found it was not there at all. The lesson is that there is no substitute for knowledge.

It took five more years before we had the second surveillance system, which was in 1955 for polio; and two more years for the third, in 1957, for influenza.

An important aspect of surveillance is that it is important to try to think from the point of view of the agent – rather like the FBI says it now does with serial killers. In December 1966, I was in Africa on a smallpox outbreak in a remote area, and we found out that we were not going to be able to get sufficient supplies of vaccine. That night, we sat

213

around a kerosene lamp and asked the question, 'What would we do if we were smallpox viruses bent on immortality?'

We communicated by radio with missionaries in the area, divided the area up so that each had a patch, asked them to send runners to every village, and twenty-four hours later we actually had a spot map. We knew which villages had smallpox. So we were able to make the best use of the small amount of vaccine we had, giving first priority to those villages. Next, we asked about market patterns and family patterns, and we chose three places that we expected smallpox to travel to. We did not know it, but it was already incubating in two of the three places. By the time the first clinical cases appeared, everyone had been vaccinated and there was no place for it to go. Smallpox disappeared in four weeks' time with just a fraction of the people actually vaccinated.

It is important to think like an agent in order to get a different perspective. The baseball player Yogi Berra once faced a new pitcher, who threw three wild pitches in a row. Berra tried for each one and missed, so with three strikes, he went back to the dugout and muttered, 'How does a pitcher like that stay in this league?' One gets a different perspective from the other side.

Another aspect of surveillance: be willing to do heroic things. It will be different for every problem, but in 1974–5, we actually decided to get rid of smallpox in India and we realized that we would actually have to go to every house. And so every three months we went to 100 million houses in a six-day period. The logistics are unbelievable: over 100 000 people doing the searching, and still more people doing the supervising evaluation. But smallpox went from the highest rates that India had had to zero in twelve months' time.

Surveillance systems can be set up very quickly. In 1955 with the Cutter incident, polio surveillance was actually initiated in the United States overnight, and was able within a period of days to show that this was a vaccine problem, but not a problem of all polio vaccines. But although surveillance systems can be set up very quickly, this is not a mode of operation we should come to depend on.

Finally, in surveillance, one should have constant feedback. One of the great examples of this is measles in the United States. Fifteen years ago, we made the decision to see if we could interrupt measles' transmission. Many people thought that we should not try because they thought it could not be done and that the effort would diminish the credibility of public health. But we decided that there was no way to know what the ultimate barriers were unless we chose the ultimate objective. And it was truly like peeling an onion. First, we found that much of the measles in the United States was being spread by military recruits who went for training, and then back home on furlough. The military quickly solved this by simply vaccinating all military recruits. Then we found there was a problem with college students, so we added college students; then with pre-schools, and so forth. Then we finally got to small problems like the Drum and Bugle Corps that would move around the country, the gypsy wedding in Spokane, one thing after another: every time we found a problem, we came up with a solution.

Now we know, because we can sequence every islet, that we have interrupted measles in the United States at least three times – and that all the measles cases we have right now are due to importation. Obviously, the way to protect American children is to get rid of measles in the world.

Another part of the problem definition is the lesson that we have learned with the EIS program, the Epidemic Intelligence Service program in the United States. This program was started as a response to the fear of biological warfare, the fear of Korean Hemorrhagic Fever. This program had had limited use in biological warfare, but as part of the training of the personnel, we learned a great deal about polio, measles and hepatitis and the problems of disease control in the United States. It helped to solve those problems because it provided us with a national network which has strengthened the public health system. I think it is one of the most important things that enabled CDC to provide consultation to people in the field. It recruited some very good people into public health who would not have gone in otherwise, and it established a new pride in public health.

The second major area is the need for a global approach, the need for global coalitions, globalization. I cannot emphasize this enough. Einstein once said that nationalism is an infantile disease, the measles of mankind, and we have to keep remembering that. There has to be a global approach, so that we no longer ask, 'How big is the problem?' It must now be, 'How big is the global problem, and how do we contribute?'

Consider smallpox, polio and Guinea worm. Our successes in all of these cases have required the WHO; but none of them came about through WHO leadership. None of these were suggested by WHO, they came because of coalitions that forced them onto the world agenda. This is such an important lesson: you cannot undertake these tasks without the World Health Organization, but do not expect them to provide the leadership. It has to be a coalition. In his book *Certain Trumpets*, Gary Wills talks about different kinds of leadership. The bottom line of that work is that lots of books talk about leadership; most of them talk about followership, but very few mention that you cannot have either without a shared goal. Shared goals are the substance of leadership.

Third, a useful approach to disease eradication or control is to change the question. Instead of asking what is the scientific problem, what are the possible interventions, ask the question, 'What would we like to do and what are the barriers to getting there?' In *Recommendations of the International Task Force on Disease Eradication*, the task force looked at 94 different infectious diseases and instead of asking whether these diseases could be eradicated, the question was, what would be the barriers to eradication; what problems would have to be solved? Suddenly, this changes everything. For example, in the case of measles, the single biggest barrier is maternal antibody. If we can develop a stealth vaccine that gets by maternal antibody, goes to the germinal centre and produces antibodies so that you could vaccinate any time after birth, suddenly measles vaccination becomes possible.

Fourth is the primacy of prevention, which is the primacy of vaccines. Given the familiar problems with drugs and pesticides, versus the value of a vaccine, even short of eradication, a vaccine might be of permanent value. We simply have to put more resources into the whole area of producing vaccines, and not just producing new vaccines, but getting away from needles and syringes. There is no reason not to think of all vaccines being oral, or by nebulizers, but with no needles or syringes. There is no reason why we could not come up with heat-stable vaccines and get rid of the cold chain which is such a problem around the world. But in order to initiate the necessary research and development, vaccines have to have primacy.

Fifth, there are some generic barriers. I think one of the big barriers to disease eradication and control is the market system itself. This is not surprising when one considers that the basis of the market system is not effective use or equity or social improvement, but money. Smallpox vaccine was on the market for 170 years, polio vaccine has now been on the market for 41 years. It is not until people make a decision that there is a political priority that we get around to the market problem. One component of the issue of drug resistance is the market system. We need to face up to it, we cannot have it both ways. We cannot have a market system and logical use. And the same thing is true for vaccines. Vaccines are not sufficiently profitable to attract company investment.

A second barrier is political will because, finally, it is not our science that caused smallpox eradication, or will lead to polio eradication, or 80 per cent immunization coverage, it is political will. There are things we can do now if there is the political will. The question is how to translate what we know into political action. On the one hundredth birthday of James Thurber, the *New York Times* carried an editorial, an article written by someone who had known James Thurber. The writer recalled a party where a woman approached him, delighted to meet him, and said, 'I live in Paris now, and they translate your column into French. I think it's even funnier in French.' Thurber replied, 'It does tend to lose something in the original.' We too lose something in the original: the science does not make sense to a great many people. We have to interpret it in order to generate the appropriate political will.

The third generic barrier is social will. I will give only one example: the role of the Rotarians in polio eradication. The Rotarians changed polio totally by pushing WHO, by pushing national leaders, by becoming involved in every country. India has recently had two polio immunization days, one in December 1995 when they immunized 88 million children in one day, and one in January 1996 when they immunized 93 million children. Social will.

The sixth and final point, the problem of leadership, specifically the importance of US leadership. In the case of smallpox eradication, the US leadership was critical. The CDC made a decision to put 300 people into smallpox eradication. Smallpox was eradicated because the leadership of the CDC, which made the decision to keep a low profile and allow WHO to have the credit in the hope that it would strengthen the WHO for other things.

In the case of polio, it was US science and the American Rotary leadership which drove the campaign. For every major recent advance, it has been the US, the CDC and the Carter Center as the driving forces. In the battle against onchocerciasis, it was an American corporation, Merck, and US leadership. In fact, December 1995 was the first time the Director-General of WHO said anything about getting more eradication.

Yet despite this splendid record, the United States has very quickly lost credibility in terms of international health leadership, for two reasons. Number one, we don't pay our dues to WHO, and number two, we are seen as the world's biggest exporters of death and disease because of arms and tobacco. Against this background, it is very hard for us to provide the leadership that is needed in this area.

What are some of the things we could be doing? Mark Twain once said, 'People who don't read have no advantage over those who can't read.' A society that does not use the information available has no advantage over a society that does not have the information. We may not be able to predict the next disease organism, but we should avoid ruining our own tools.

What are some of the steps? The first one, I think, has to do with exploring ways of combining the marketplace and disease control needs. When new therapeutic agents come on the market, there should be a global protocol on how we are going to employ them. What would be the most effective way to do this? Then, how do we compensate pharmaceutical companies much as we compensate farmers, for not producing? How can we give them an honest amount of money for not just putting products out in the market? How do we keep doctors from feeling that they should be able to prescribe any drug? How do we get a group of experts for every drug who have to give approval for the use of that drug?

Could we set up such a protocol and have some people with the authority for a particular drug, and how would we get global agreement? This is going to be a tough problem, but it is one of the things we should really put the wisest people up against.

We are capable of changing and there are precedents. We have hospitals where infectious disease epidemiologists are now approving the use of antibiotics. In the past, there have been some drugs where the CDC had to give approval for national use. Could we do the same thing on a global basis?

Second, could we think through our desires in this area and then come up with what would be the perfect global surveillance system? We need a generic plan, because we do not know which agents will come up. It could include traditional surveillance of antibiotic sensitivity. This would have to be global, it would have to be for all human beings, and it would have to include animals.

We would have to put money into more rapid diagnostic techniques. It is not simply that in some areas we do not have diagnostic techniques at all. I wonder, if we did a crash program, whether we could not come up with a way to do an instantaneous diagnosis on microorganisms. I think the ability is there if we harnessed it correctly. It would include modeling. My first involvement with modeling was in the 1960s when we got Dr George McDonald of the London School, who had done all the modeling on malaria, and asked him the question, 'what would we have to do to interrupt measles under African conditions?' It turns out that measles does in fact change according to population density. The problem you encounter is in places like Lagos where the median age of measles is 14 or 15 months, which gives you almost no window between when the children lose maternal antibodies and when they contract the disease.

It would include an inventory of all the systems we now have, to bring them together and ask how to fill the gaps. This includes, of course, strengthening our own US surveillance capacity. To date, our response to this has been a weakening of the public health system in the United States. Some of it is deliberate, with the reduction of resources; some of it has come about indirectly through health care reforms.

Third, I think we should support the global equivalent of an EIS program. Fifteen years ago, Secretary Schweicher went to the World Health Assembly with such a proposal. He made an offer that the US would help WHO develop a global EIS program, but there was never a response. Yet I think it would have the same benefits of providing a way to get surveillance, a way to investigate, a way to have a global approach.

Fourth and finally, we have to exert pressure on our own political system to again have US leadership in international health. The first thing is that we simply have to pay our dues. Twelve years ago, when we were in the same position, I wrote an editorial and quoted Dolly Parton, 'You'd be surprised how much it costs to look this cheap.' And the United States is going to find out how much it costs to look this cheap. But second, then support a global EIS Program, support an international health track for the training of young people.

Recently, I spoke with a woman who was once a Peace Corps volunteer in Liberia and she told me a story about the time when the United States first put someone on the moon. When the news reached her village, the blacksmith invited her to his house, along with the men of the village. He asked, is it true that there is an American on the moon? Yes, she replied. And was it true that he was put in a rocket and sent up there? Yes, she answered. He shook his head and said, 'Those Americans, they sure are good blacksmiths.'

We certainly are good blacksmiths, and we have something to offer in infectious disease control, too. How can we get this knowledge and ability to apply to the world situation? In an editorial written twenty years ago, Norman Cousins asked the question, 'What is the single greatest gift the US has given the world in 200 years?' His answer was that our single biggest gift is the idea that it is possible to plan a rational future. Our gift to the world could be that it is possible to plan a rational health future. Are we wise enough to do that?

* This is an edited transcript of a speech given by William Foege to the Cantigny Conference, 'Strategic Implications of Global Microbial Threats', 14 June 1996.

Index